My Personal Path to Wellness

A Journal for
Living Creatively
with Chronic Illness

_____

Treena and Graham Kerr

With Chavanne Hanson, RD, LD

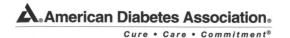

American Diabetes Association.

Cure • Care • Commitment®

Director, Book Publishing, John Fedor; *Associate Director, Consumer Books and Editor,* Sherrye Landrum; *Associate Director, Book Production,* Peggy M. Rote; *Composition,* Circle Graphics, Inc.; *Cover Design,* Koncept, Inc.; *Printer,* Port City Press.

Printed in the United States of America

1 3 5 7 9 10 8 6 4 2

The suggestions and information contained in this publication are generally consistent with the *Clinical Practice Recommendations* and other policies of the American Diabetes Association, but they do not represent the policy or position of the Association or any of its boards or committees. Reasonable steps have been taken to ensure the accuracy of the information presented. However, the American Diabetes Association cannot ensure the safety or efficacy of any product or service described in this publication. Individuals are advised to consult a physician or other appropriate health care professional before undertaking any diet or exercise program or taking any medication referred to in this publication. Professionals must use and apply their own professional judgment, experience, and training and should not rely solely on the information contained in this publication before prescribing any diet, exercise, or medication. The American Diabetes Association—its officers, directors, employees, volunteers, and members—assumes no responsibility or liability for personal or other injury, loss, or damage that may result from the suggestions or information in this publication.

♾ The paper in this publication meets the requirements of the ANSI Standard Z39.48-1992 (permanence of paper).

ADA titles may be purchased for business or promotional use or for special sales. To purchase this book in large quantities, or for custom editions of this book with your logo, contact Lee Romano Sequeira, Special Sales & Promotions, at the address below, or at LRomano@diabetes.org or 703-299-2046.

American Diabetes Association
1701 North Beauregard Street
Alexandria, Virginia 22311

Library of Congress Cataloging-in-Publication Data

Kerr, Treena, 1934–
 My personal path to wellness: a journal for living creatively with chronic illness / Treena and Graham Kerr.
   p. cm.
 ISBN 1-58040-214-3 (pbk: alk. paper)
 1. Diabetes—Popular works. 2. Coronary heart disease—Popular works. 3. Diaries (Blank-books) 4. Self-care, Health. I. Kerr, Graham. II. Title.

RC660.4.K473 2004
616.1'230654—dc22   2004045069

Contents

Acknowledgments

Throughout this journal is sprinkled the wisdom of nearly one hundred health professionals who strongly believe in *evidence* based lifestyle suggestions. Each contributor has been a guest on our TV show *The Gathering Place*, which is shown nationwide. Our very own resident scientist Chavanne Hanson, RD, has carefully selected more than three hundred of their suggestions and included them as "ideas in season" throughout the journal.

To each of you that so enthusiastically contributed to our knowledge of what constitutes good health, we say a warm "thank you." We have gained mightily by knowing you and by absorbing and making direct application of your wisdom.

And thank you once again, Chavanne, for all the years you have so faithfully guided us in our search for evidence based lifestyle alternatives.

And Sherrye, where would we be without your love and laughter and depth of commitment to the reader?

Thank you again, everyone.
Graham and Treena Kerr

Introduction

Treena and I could not be more delighted!

e have quite literally prayed that you would decide to "journal" your way to wellness . . . and that you would read this brief introduction. So, we are doubly delighted!

This journal is based upon the journals and charts that we've kept together for the past 15 years. We've kept these records (at first sketchily) since our lifestyle trial in Hawaii when our cardiologist gave us three months to see what effect the dietary and exercise changes would have on Treena's 365 mg/dl cholesterol following her stroke and heart attack.

You tend to keep a good track record when the alternative is open heart surgery!

We've gradually adjusted our process, and today, we (and our care team) can see at a glance exactly how we are doing. On these pages, you can note everything from the water you drink to how you felt and what your blood sugar was at any time of day. The carbohydrate (carb) count in your meals is set out because it affects your blood sugar the most. Along the bottom are icons you X out for the veggies, fruits, nuts, and whole grains you've eaten that day. When you add fruit, vegetables, and whole grains to your meals, you get nutrients and fiber that your body needs. Nuts and seeds provide healthy fats our bodies need and may have been missing with the craze of low-fat diets. Olive and canola oil also supply good fats. We sprinkle freshly ground flaxseed on our morning cereal to get the omega-3 fats that our hearts need.

Our success is based on checking, recording, and using the numbers to rate lifestyle adjustments. We check Treena's blood glucose two hours after the first bite of the meal to see how her blood sugar reacts to a new recipe or an adjusted one. We use fasting blood glucose to check on daily trends and to see the effects of exercise, stress, travel, pain, and sick days as well as bouts of depression.

We chart daily numbers on a monthly chart, another way to see trends and look for causes. We keep a monthly record of blood sugar levels, blood pressure, and weight. You could also record weekly blood sugar averages and cholesterol levels to see them improve.

I (Graham) feel pretty sure that you may think charting *all* this information could border on obsessive compulsive, but I don't. We do it to be full partners with our physician, our diabetes educator, and our cardiologist in Treena's future health. Treena chooses every day to measure her progress. We can spot a negative trend before it takes hold and see an improvement and understand what we did that was right.

We call this journal our Daily Olympics of Life (DOOL). By this name, we acknowledge the *fact* that we must chart a careful course between a rock (heart disease) and a hard place (diabetes). So far, we have avoided diabetes complications. Treena's AlC drop from 11.9 to 6.1 represents a 6 point drop, which experts regard as a 180% drop in risk factors for another stroke or heart attack. The whole story and 430 recipes for you to make your own can be found in our *Charting a Course to Wellness: Creative Ways of Living with Heart Disease and Diabetes* (ADA, 2004).

Our journey to wellness is an ongoing voyage that we choose to embrace and celebrate with an overwhelming sense of gratitude. We know where we've been—day by day—and we have information to help us choose the next direction to take. Our destination is secure.

Now you have the tool to chart your journey. Please consider keeping a daily log and most importantly, share your progress with the one you love.

With all our love and prayers,
Graham and Treena Kerr

What to Think about as You Keep Your Journal

| Date _____ Deep Breathing _____ Sleep _____ |
| HOURS |

Water ☐ ☐ ☐ ☐ ☐ ☐ ☐ ☐   Blood Pressure _____

F O O D

BREAKFAST   Time   Total Carb _____

       Serving Size   Food and Drinks

Grain
Vegetable
Protein
Fruit
Milk
Fat

SNACK   Time   Total Carb _____

LUNCH   Time   Total Carb _____

       Serving Size   Food and Drinks

Grain
Vegetable
Protein
Fruit
Milk
Fat

SNACK   Time   Total Carb _____

DINNER   Time   Total Carb _____

       Serving Size   Food and Drinks

Grain
Vegetable
Protein
Fruit
Milk
Fat

TOTALS

VEGETABLES   FRUIT   NUTS   WHOLE GRAINS

First Page

Take a few minutes to familiarize yourself with the different sections of the journal page. You will see that we begin with the absolute basics—air, water, and sleep. We recommend that everyone stop and spend at least five minutes every day just breathing deeply. It relieves stress and makes you feel good. Just cross off the number of glasses of water you drink. Glasses of tea count here, but not soda or juice—too much sugar. Water keeps you healthier and helps your medications work as they're supposed to. There's a place to record your blood pressure, if you have a blood pressure cuff for at-home checks.

Food is a big category, so it gets more room for details. You can just check off the different food groups. You can write in the food and serving size (which is really important). For those with diabetes, the carb count of the meal is important for predicting the rise in blood sugar that follows in about two hours. Or you can count carbs for losing weight.

At the bottom of the page, the little icons for vegetables, fruit, nuts, and whole grains give you a quick way to track how you're meeting the goals of adding fruits, vegetables, and whole grains to your meals. The nut icon stands for healthy fats found in nuts, seeds, and olives, avocados, and olive and canola oils. If you include 3 servings of vegetables, 2 servings of fruit, and 2 servings of healthy fats in your daily meals, you'll make a difference in how you feel, what you weigh, and how healthy your heart is!

You don't have to fill in all the sections every day. But the more you fill in, the better you come to know yourself. If you are tracking a lifestyle change, practice it for 90 days, and it will become part of who you are—the new, healthier, wiser you.

Second Page

We are emotional and spiritual beings, too, and these parts of us affect our physical health. You may just want to track your energy level—it's a true measure of the effect of better food choices and regular exercise on you. We also include a chart for checking on your emotions at the end of this introduction and then at the end of the daily charts, so you can see what has changed.

We have spaces for all kinds of physical fun: aerobic exercise to work heart, lungs, and body in the "walking" line; weights or resistance exercises; stretches, and so on. You need variety to get the most benefits. Your weight rests in this section, because muscle—which you build with exercise—burns calories even at rest!

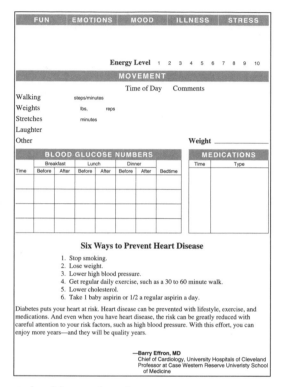

Those of you with diabetes can use the next section for blood glucose numbers. Most people with type 2 diabetes check before breakfast—a fasting glucose. Choose one other time of day and vary it between before and after meals. If you've eaten more carb than usual, or a new recipe, you might want to check 2 hours after the first bite to see what happens.

The medications section can apply to anyone, but is attached to the blood glucose record because most people with diabetes take oral meds or insulin, and may also take cholesterol or blood pressure medication. We hope you have enough room to record them here.

The next section holds tips from the health professional guests on our TV show. You may notice a pattern to what they say, and we hope you do. The truth is the truth is the truth.

In the back of the book are charts that can show trends in each month, so you can try to figure out the causes . . . for example, the effect a business trip or illness has on your weight or blood sugar. Knowing that change comes in small steps, we've included menu charts and an activity planner to help you make changes on paper before you try them in real life.

Women, Diabetes, and Cardiovascular Disease

Women with diabetes are at high risk for having heart disease or a stroke. In fact, two of three women with diabetes die from heart disease or stroke. But the good news is that you can delay or prevent problems by managing the ABCs of diabetes.

A Is for A1C

An A-1-C is the blood glucose check with a memory. It tells you your average blood glucose for the past 2–3 months. The American Diabetes Association (ADA) recommends that most people aim for an A1C below 7. Talk with your health care provider about the best target for you.

B Is for Blood Pressure

Your blood pressure numbers tell you the force of blood inside your blood vessels. It's like the pressure of water in a garden hose. When your blood pressure is high, your heart has to work harder than it should. The ADA recommends that you keep your blood pressure below 130/80 (130 over 80).

C Is for Cholesterol

Your cholesterol numbers tell you the amount of fat in your blood. Some kinds of fat, such as HDL cholesterol, help protect your heart. Other kinds, such as LDL cholesterol, can clog your blood vessels and lead to heart disease. Triglycerides are another kind of blood fat that raises your risk for heart disease. The chart below gives the targets suggested by the ADA.

ADA TARGETS		MY RESULTS	
		Date	Numbers
A1C	Below 7%		
Blood pressure	Below 130/80 mmHg		
LDL cholesterol	Below 100 mg/dl		
HDL cholesterol	Above 50 mg/dl		
Triglycerides	Below 150 mg/dl		

Emotions

Here is a little list of emotions . . . really our general feelings about our life and how we are living it in our heads and hearts. You can fill it in now and then again later in the year. We've given you another chart like this at the end of the daily charts. Fill it in and compare it to when you began. It's such fun to see progress! Simply check the number after the feelings that best describe how you feel *TODAY*.

I'M GRATEFUL FOR THESE

Loving	1	2	3	4	5	6	7	8	9	10
Joyful	1	2	3	4	5	6	7	8	9	10
Peaceful	1	2	3	4	5	6	7	8	9	10
Patient	1	2	3	4	5	6	7	8	9	10
Gentle	1	2	3	4	5	6	7	8	9	10
Ethical	1	2	3	4	5	6	7	8	9	10
Faithful	1	2	3	4	5	6	7	8	9	10
Mild Mannered	1	2	3	4	5	6	7	8	9	10
Self Controlled	1	2	3	4	5	6	7	8	9	10

I'M WORKING ON THESE

Resentment	1	2	3	4	5	6	7	8	9	10
Despondent	1	2	3	4	5	6	7	8	9	10
Argumentative	1	2	3	4	5	6	7	8	9	10
Impatient	1	2	3	4	5	6	7	8	9	10
Impetuous	1	2	3	4	5	6	7	8	9	10
Abusive (Hurtful)	1	2	3	4	5	6	7	8	9	10
Unreliable	1	2	3	4	5	6	7	8	9	10
Conceited (Vain)	1	2	3	4	5	6	7	8	9	10
Dissatisfied	1	2	3	4	5	6	7	8	9	10

(1 = Less; 10 = More Obvious)

Daily Journal Pages

*T*hink about where you would like to be—or maybe who you would like to be—four months from now . . . what you want to look like, what you want to be doing, the new lifestyle habits you want to be yours.

Along the way it might help to think about how you feel about having a chronic disease . . . or do you want to prevent one from developing? A disease can be—as it was for us—the motivation for changing yourself to be more like the person you wish you were! Here is a tool for translating your wishes into actions.

Our bodies are miracle machines that respond quickly to loving care from us, the owners. Your health is measured in physical, mental, emotional, and spiritual dimensions. When you realize this, you are rich as well as wise.

DATE: _____

My weight today is _____.

My blood pressure is _____.

My LDL (bad) cholesterol is _____.

My HDL (good) cholesterol is _____.

My triglyceride level is _____.

My AIC is _____.

My BG level is _____.

Date __2-25-04__ Deep Breathing __10 minutes__ Sleep __8__
HOURS
Water ☒ ☒ ☒ ☒ ☐ ☐ ☐ ☐ Blood Pressure __120/82__

F O O D

BREAKFAST Time __8:30 am__ Total Carb __65 g__

	Serving Size	Food and Drinks	
Grain	1 c.	cereal	30 g
Vegetable			
Protein			
Fruit	2 slices	pineapple	20 g
Milk	1 8-oz glass	milk	15 g
Fat	6	almonds	

SNACK Time __10:45__ Total Carb __15 g__

17	grapes

LUNCH Time __12:30__ Total Carb __75 g__

	Serving Size	Food and Drinks	
Grain	1 6-in	pita bread, whole wheat	30 g
Vegetable	2 c.	lettuce, tomato, mushrooms, red bell pepper	30 g
Protein	2 oz	chopped chicken breast	
Fruit	3/4 c.	mandarin oranges	15 g
Milk			
Fat	2 T.	reduced fat salad dressing	

SNACK Time __3:20__ Total Carb __10 g__

1/4 c.	trail mix: raisins, nuts, and dried fruit

DINNER Time __6:00__ Total Carb __68 g__

	Serving Size	Food and Drinks	
Grain	2/3 cups	Brown rice	30 g
Vegetable	1	sliced tomato on lettuce	15 g
Protein	1 serving	Pepper stead	8 g
Fruit	1 small	baked apple	15 g
Milk			
Fat	1 T.	olice oil on tomato	

T O T A L S

VEGETABLES ☒☒☒☒ FRUIT ☒☒ NUTS ☒☒ WHOLE GRAINS ☒

FUN	EMOTIONS	MOOD	ILLNESS	STRESS
sang and danced to favorite CD	excited about the trip worried about Dr's appt.	so-so	scratchy throat	packing for a trip

Energy Level   1   2   3   4   5   (6)   7   8   9   10

MOVEMENT

		Time of Day	Comments
Walking	_30 min._ steps/minutes	3:30	enjoyed the sun & strong breeze
Weights	_3_ lbs, _15_ reps x 3	4:00	found I could do another set
Stretches	_15_ minutes	4:45	of reps today!
Laughter	_5 minutes in a.m. 30 + in p.m._		
Other	_walked the dog 4 times today_		**Weight** _122_

BLOOD GLUCOSE NUMBERS

Time	Breakfast Before	Breakfast After	Lunch Before	Lunch After	Dinner Before	Dinner After	Bedtime
7 a.m.	90						
2:00				152			
6 p.m.					100		
9:30							120

MEDICATIONS

Time	Type
7:00 a.m.	statin
7:00 a.m.	Glucophage
6:30 p.m.	Glucophage

Six Ways to Prevent Heart Disease

1. Stop smoking.
2. Lose weight.
3. Lower high blood pressure.
4. Get regular daily exercise, such as a 30 to 60 minute walk.
5. Lower cholesterol.
6. Take 1 baby aspirin or 1/2 a regular aspirin a day.

Diabetes puts your heart at risk. Heart disease can be prevented with lifestyle, exercise, and medications. And even when you have heart disease, the risk can be greatly reduced with careful attention to your risk factors, such as high blood pressure. With this effort, you can enjoy more years—and they will be quality years.

—**Barry Effron, MD**
Chief of Cardiology, University Hospitals of Cleveland
Professor at Case Western Reserve University School of Medicine

Date _____ Deep Breathing _____ Sleep _____

HOURS

Water ⊔ ⊔ ⊔ ⊔ ⊔ ⊔ ⊔ ⊔   Blood Pressure _____

F O O D

BREAKFAST   Time _____ Total Carb_____

         Serving Size   Food and Drinks

Grain

Vegetable

Protein

Fruit

Milk

Fat

SNACK   Time _____ Total Carb_____

LUNCH   Time _____ Total Carb_____

         Serving Size   Food and Drinks

Grain

Vegetable

Protein

Fruit

Milk

Fat

SNACK   Time _____ Total Carb_____

DINNER   Time _____ Total Carb_____

         Serving Size   Food and Drinks

Grain

Vegetable

Protein

Fruit

Milk

Fat

TOTALS

VEGETABLES   FRUIT   NUTS   WHOLE GRAINS

Energy Level 1 2 3 4 5 6 7 8 9 10

MOVEMENT

Time of Day   Comments

Walking _____ steps/minutes

Weights _____ lbs, _____ reps

Stretches _____ minutes

Laughter _____

Other _____   **Weight** _____

BLOOD GLUCOSE NUMBERS

Time	Breakfast		Lunch		Dinner		Bedtime
	Before	After	Before	After	Before	After	

MEDICATIONS

Time	Type

Six Ways to Prevent Heart Disease

1. Stop smoking.
2. Lose weight.
3. Lower high blood pressure.
4. Get regular daily exercise, such as a 30 to 60 minute walk.
5. Lower cholesterol.
6. Take 1 baby aspirin or 1/2 a regular aspirin a day.

Diabetes puts your heart at risk. Heart disease can be prevented with lifestyle, exercise, and medications. And even when you have heart disease, the risk can be greatly reduced with careful attention to your risk factors, such as high blood pressure. With this effort, you can enjoy more years—and they will be quality years.

—Barry Effron, MD
Chief of Cardiology, University Hospitals of Cleveland
Professor at Case Western Reserve University School of Medicine

Date _____ Deep Breathing _____ Sleep _____

Water ⎕ ⎕ ⎕ ⎕ ⎕ ⎕ ⎕ ⎕   HOURS

Blood Pressure _____

FOOD

BREAKFAST Time _____ Total Carb_____

	Serving Size	Food and Drinks
Grain		
Vegetable		
Protein		
Fruit		
Milk		
Fat		

SNACK Time _____ Total Carb_____

LUNCH Time _____ Total Carb_____

	Serving Size	Food and Drinks
Grain		
Vegetable		
Protein		
Fruit		
Milk		
Fat		

SNACK Time _____ Total Carb_____

DINNER Time _____ Total Carb_____

	Serving Size	Food and Drinks
Grain		
Vegetable		
Protein		
Fruit		
Milk		
Fat		

TOTALS

VEGETABLES   FRUIT   NUTS   WHOLE GRAINS

FUN	EMOTIONS	MOOD	ILLNESS	STRESS

Energy Level 1 2 3 4 5 6 7 8 9 10

MOVEMENT

Time of Day   Comments

Walking _____ steps/minutes

Weights _____ lbs, _____ reps

Stretches _____ minutes

Laughter _____

Other _____ **Weight** _____

BLOOD GLUCOSE NUMBERS						
	Breakfast		Lunch		Dinner	
Time	Before	After	Before	After	Before	After	Bedtime

MEDICATIONS	
Time	Type

Healthy Insight for the Day

GRAHAM

A daily journal can help you track the food you eat, exercise, test results, sleep schedule, weight, and other measurements. It is the only way you can see where you are, what you actually do, and when you make changes, how you are progressing with them. A journal is a great way to track accomplishments and stay focused on your goals.

Date _____ Deep Breathing _____ Sleep _____

Water ☐ ☐ ☐ ☐ ☐ ☐ ☐ ☐   Blood Pressure _____

HOURS

F O O D

BREAKFAST
Time _____ Total Carb_____

Serving Size	Food and Drinks

Grain
Vegetable
Protein
Fruit
Milk
Fat

SNACK
Time _____ Total Carb_____

LUNCH
Time _____ Total Carb_____

Serving Size	Food and Drinks

Grain
Vegetable
Protein
Fruit
Milk
Fat

SNACK
Time _____ Total Carb_____

DINNER
Time _____ Total Carb_____

Serving Size	Food and Drinks

Grain
Vegetable
Protein
Fruit
Milk
Fat

T O T A L S

VEGETABLES   FRUIT   NUTS   WHOLE GRAINS

FUN	EMOTIONS	MOOD	ILLNESS	STRESS

Energy Level 1 2 3 4 5 6 7 8 9 10

MOVEMENT

Time of Day Comments

Walking _____ steps/minutes

Weights _____ lbs, _____ reps

Stretches _____ minutes

Laughter _____

Other _____ **Weight** _____

BLOOD GLUCOSE NUMBERS

Time	Breakfast		Lunch		Dinner		Bedtime
	Before	After	Before	After	Before	After	

MEDICATIONS

Time	Type

Whole Grains

Whole grains are a powerhouse of nutrition, providing the energy your body loves and vitamins, minerals, and fiber. Here's more about whole grains:

- Choose from a wealth of grains: amaranth, millet, quinoa, couscous, bulgur, cracked wheat, barley, buckwheat, brown rice, Scottish oats.
- Add grains to dishes for taste and texture: soups, stews, chilies, salads, casseroles.
- Use whole grains for special occasions, such as stuffing at holiday times.
- Each month, buy a whole grain you have never tried before.
- The first ingredient on the ingredients list should be whole wheat, whole oats, or whole barley. The key is that the word "whole" appears before the grain.
- Refrigerate or freeze whole grains or whole grain flours to keep them from going rancid.

—Judi Adams, MS, RD
President, Wheat Foods Council

Date _____ Deep Breathing _____ Sleep _____

HOURS

Water ☐ ☐ ☐ ☐ ☐ ☐ ☐ ☐   Blood Pressure _____

F O O D

BREAKFAST
Time _____ Total Carb_____

Serving Size   Food and Drinks

Grain
Vegetable
Protein
Fruit
Milk
Fat

SNACK
Time _____ Total Carb_____

LUNCH
Time _____ Total Carb_____

Serving Size   Food and Drinks

Grain
Vegetable
Protein
Fruit
Milk
Fat

SNACK
Time _____ Total Carb_____

DINNER
Time _____ Total Carb_____

Serving Size   Food and Drinks

Grain
Vegetable
Protein
Fruit
Milk
Fat

T O T A L S

VEGETABLES   FRUIT   NUTS   WHOLE GRAINS

FUN	EMOTIONS	MOOD	ILLNESS	STRESS

Energy Level 1 2 3 4 5 6 7 8 9 10

MOVEMENT

Time of Day   Comments

Walking _____ steps/minutes

Weights _____ lbs, _____ reps

Stretches _____ minutes

Laughter _____

Other _____   **Weight** _____

BLOOD GLUCOSE NUMBERS

Time	Breakfast		Lunch		Dinner		Bedtime
	Before	After	Before	After	Before	After	

MEDICATIONS

Time	Type

Self Hearing Test

Yes = 4, Sometimes = 2, No = 0

If you score more than 10, have your hearing checked by a doctor.

1. Do you feel embarrassed when meeting new people because you can't hear their names?
2. Does your hearing cause you to feel frustrated when talking to members of your family? Or frustrate them when talking to you?
3. Do you have difficulty hearing when someone speaks in a whisper?
4. Do you feel handicapped about a hearing problem?
5. Is your hearing a problem when you visit friends, relatives, or neighbors?
6. Is your hearing a problem at movies, the theatre, or religious services?
7. Does your hearing cause you to have arguments with family members?
8. Does your hearing make it difficult to listen to the television or radio?
9. Do you feel that your hearing limits your personal or social style?
10. Is your hearing a problem in a restaurant with relatives or friends?

—Steve Allen, MD
State University of New York Health Sciences, Syracuse

Date _____ Deep Breathing _____ Sleep _____
HOURS

Water ▢ ▢ ▢ ▢ ▢ ▢ ▢ ▢   Blood Pressure _____

F O O D

BREAKFAST　　　　　　Time _____ Total Carb_____

　　　　Serving Size　　Food and Drinks

Grain
Vegetable
Protein
Fruit
Milk
Fat

SNACK　　　　　　　　Time _____ Total Carb_____

LUNCH　　　　　　　　Time _____ Total Carb_____

　　　　Serving Size　　Food and Drinks

Grain
Vegetable
Protein
Fruit
Milk
Fat

SNACK　　　　　　　　Time _____ Total Carb_____

DINNER　　　　　　　　Time _____ Total Carb_____

　　　　Serving Size　　Food and Drinks

Grain
Vegetable
Protein
Fruit
Milk
Fat

T O T A L S

VEGETABLES　　　　FRUIT　　　NUTS　　　WHOLE GRAINS

FUN	EMOTIONS	MOOD	ILLNESS	STRESS

Energy Level   1   2   3   4   5   6   7   8   9   10

MOVEMENT

Time of Day   Comments

Walking _____ steps/minutes

Weights _____ lbs, _____ reps

Stretches _____ minutes

Laughter _____

Other _____   **Weight** _____

BLOOD GLUCOSE NUMBERS

Time	Breakfast		Lunch		Dinner		Bedtime
	Before	After	Before	After	Before	After	

MEDICATIONS

Time	Type

Top Healing Herbs and the Reported Benefits

Garlic: antibiotic; lowers cholesterol and high blood pressure; seems to be better for you raw, so try chopping it up, mixing with a bit of honey and swallow—should be no odor.

Thyme: decongestant herb, germ killing.

Ginger: stops motion sickness and settles the stomach.

Peppermint: relieve gas and indigestion.

Fennel Seeds: helps digestion and is good for your breath, good for baby's colic.

Using herbal remedies can be healing because you are taking control of your health. Get guidance from your health care provider and be cautious with the amount you consume. Just as with medications, large doses of some herbs can be toxic and harmful.

—**Sara Altshul O'Donnell**
Alternative Medicine Editor, *Prevention* magazine

Date _____ Deep Breathing _____ Sleep _____
                                                                    HOURS

Water 🥛 🥛 🥛 🥛 🥛 🥛 🥛 🥛   Blood Pressure _____

F O O D

BREAKFAST   Time _____ Total Carb_____

      Serving Size   Food and Drinks
Grain
Vegetable
Protein
Fruit
Milk
Fat

_____

SNACK   Time _____ Total Carb_____

_____

LUNCH   Time _____ Total Carb_____

      Serving Size   Food and Drinks
Grain
Vegetable
Protein
Fruit
Milk
Fat

_____

SNACK   Time _____ Total Carb_____

_____

DINNER   Time _____ Total Carb_____

      Serving Size   Food and Drinks
Grain
Vegetable
Protein
Fruit
Milk
Fat

_____

T O T A L S

VEGETABLES   FRUIT   NUTS   WHOLE GRAINS

FUN	EMOTIONS	MOOD	ILLNESS	STRESS

Energy Level 1 2 3 4 5 6 7 8 9 10

MOVEMENT

Time of Day   Comments

Walking _____ steps/minutes

Weights _____ lbs, _____ reps

Stretches _____ minutes

Laughter _____

Other _____ **Weight** _____

BLOOD GLUCOSE NUMBERS

Time	Breakfast Before	Breakfast After	Lunch Before	Lunch After	Dinner Before	Dinner After	Bedtime

MEDICATIONS

Time	Type

Tea

If you are looking for a tasty alternative to sodas, try tea. The benefits are many, especially for your immune system. To prepare herbal teas:

- Put the herbs in an infuser, tea bag, or tea ball (1 tsp herb per cup of water)
- Boil fresh water in a teakettle, and pour over the herbs in a teapot
- Keep pot covered, and let it steep 10–15 minutes (or as directed)
  Green teas should only steep about 2 minutes or they get bitter.
- Spices in your spice rack that can be good teas include thyme, garlic, and any aromatic herb that smells good
- Roots and woody herbs take longer to steep

White, green, and black tea all come from the same plant, and all contain antioxidants to help you stay healthy. Red tea (rooibos from South Africa) comes from a different plant but has 50% more antioxidants than black tea.

—Sara Altshul O'Donnell
Alternative Medicine Editor, *Prevention* magazine

Date _____ Deep Breathing _____ Sleep _____
HOURS

Water ☐ ☐ ☐ ☐ ☐ ☐ ☐ ☐   Blood Pressure _____

F O O D

BREAKFAST Time _____ Total Carb_____

	Serving Size	Food and Drinks
Grain		
Vegetable		
Protein		
Fruit		
Milk		
Fat		

SNACK Time _____ Total Carb_____

LUNCH Time _____ Total Carb_____

	Serving Size	Food and Drinks
Grain		
Vegetable		
Protein		
Fruit		
Milk		
Fat		

SNACK Time _____ Total Carb_____

DINNER Time _____ Total Carb_____

	Serving Size	Food and Drinks
Grain		
Vegetable		
Protein		
Fruit		
Milk		
Fat		

T O T A L S

VEGETABLES   FRUIT   NUTS   WHOLE GRAINS

FUN	EMOTIONS	MOOD	ILLNESS	STRESS

Energy Level 1 2 3 4 5 6 7 8 9 10

MOVEMENT

Time of Day   Comments

Walking _____ steps/minutes

Weights _____ lbs, _____ reps

Stretches _____ minutes

Laughter _____

Other _____   **Weight** _____

BLOOD GLUCOSE NUMBERS							
Time	Breakfast		Lunch		Dinner		Bedtime
	Before	After	Before	After	Before	After	

MEDICATIONS	
Time	Type

Diabetes

Type 1 diabetes comes on rapidly and usually in young people. They need insulin immediately. Symptoms of extreme thirst, frequent urination, and fatigue go away with insulin. **Type 2 diabetes** strikes 90% of people with diabetes. People at risk, even children, often have warning signs such as: overweight, high blood pressure, family history, being in certain ethnic groups, and having had a large baby.

You have diabetes if your fasting blood glucose on two different days is above 126 mg/dl. At 110–125 mg/dl, you have pre-diabetes, and it's time to change your lifestyle. Normal blood sugar is 80–120 mg/dl before meals.

What Affects Blood Sugar?

Food

Activity

Insulin

Stress (illness, tension, hormone swings)

—Richard S. Beaser, MD
Joslin Diabetes Center

Date _____ Deep Breathing _____ Sleep _____
                                                                        HOURS

Water ⬜ ⬜ ⬜ ⬜ ⬜ ⬜ ⬜ ⬜   Blood Pressure _____

FOOD

BREAKFAST   Time _____ Total Carb_____

　　　　Serving Size   Food and Drinks
Grain
Vegetable
Protein
Fruit
Milk
Fat

SNACK   Time _____ Total Carb_____

LUNCH   Time _____ Total Carb_____

　　　　Serving Size   Food and Drinks
Grain
Vegetable
Protein
Fruit
Milk
Fat

SNACK   Time _____ Total Carb_____

DINNER   Time _____ Total Carb_____

　　　　Serving Size   Food and Drinks
Grain
Vegetable
Protein
Fruit
Milk
Fat

TOTALS

VEGETABLES   FRUIT   NUTS   WHOLE GRAINS

Energy Level 1 2 3 4 5 6 7 8 9 10

MOVEMENT

Time of Day   Comments

Walking _____ steps/minutes

Weights _____ lbs, _____ reps

Stretches _____ minutes

Laughter _____

Other _____

Weight _____

BLOOD GLUCOSE NUMBERS

| Time | Breakfast | | Lunch | | Dinner | | Bedtime |
	Before	After	Before	After	Before	After	

MEDICATIONS

Time	Type

Why Are So Many Children Obese?

- Children are less active than ever before, so they don't burn the calories they eat.
- Busy lifestyles lead to fast food (high in calories and fat) as a regular meal for kids—even at school.
- Children learn from their parents' example. If parents have poor eating habits, the children will, too.
- Infants who always have a bottle handy may be overfed, starting obesity early. Fruit juice is sugar water just as much as soda is.
- Children are taught to eat everything on the plate, even though they know when they are full and want to stop eating.
- Children have problems when indulgent parents or grandparents serve a lot of high calorie food that "must be eaten."

—Glenn Berall, MD
Chief of Pediatrics, Toronto Western Hospital

Date _____ Deep Breathing _____ Sleep _____
                                                             HOURS

Water ⊔ ⊔ ⊔ ⊔ ⊔ ⊔ ⊔ ⊔   Blood Pressure _____

F O O D

BREAKFAST   Time _____ Total Carb_____

        Serving Size   Food and Drinks

Grain
Vegetable
Protein
Fruit
Milk
Fat

SNACK   Time _____ Total Carb_____

LUNCH   Time _____ Total Carb_____

        Serving Size   Food and Drinks

Grain
Vegetable
Protein
Fruit
Milk
Fat

SNACK   Time _____ Total Carb_____

DINNER   Time _____ Total Carb_____

        Serving Size   Food and Drinks

Grain
Vegetable
Protein
Fruit
Milk
Fat

T O T A L S

VEGETABLES   FRUIT   NUTS   WHOLE GRAINS

| FUN | EMOTIONS | MOOD | ILLNESS | STRESS |

Energy Level 1   2   3   4   5   6   7   8   9   10

MOVEMENT

Time of Day   Comments

Walking _____ steps/minutes

Weights _____ lbs, _____ reps

Stretches _____ minutes

Laughter _____

Other _____   **Weight** _____

BLOOD GLUCOSE NUMBERS							
	Breakfast		Lunch		Dinner		
Time	Before	After	Before	After	Before	After	Bedtime

MEDICATIONS	
Time	Type

Protein

If you don't eat, muscle tissue is burned for fuel, not fat. Muscle weighs more than fat, so you see rapid weight loss, but you've still got the unhealthy fat.

- Our bodies use protein to build and repair tissues, hormones, enzymes, hair, skin, and to keep the heart beating—in short, for everything.
- Protein comes from animals and plants, including chicken, fish, cheese, dairy products, eggs, meat, nuts, beans, and soy.
- Protein is made of 22 amino acids. To get them all from plant proteins, eat two or more in the same day.
- Too much protein stresses the kidneys with ketones and toxins. Muscle tissue is torn down rather than built up. You build muscles with weight training, not by eating lots of protein.
- Too little protein causes the body to break down its muscle mass to get the amino acids it needs.

—Jacqueline Berning, PhD, RD
Assistant Professor at University of Colorado

Date _____ Deep Breathing _____ Sleep _____

Water ▢ ▢ ▢ ▢ ▢ ▢ ▢ ▢   Blood Pressure _____

HOURS

F O O D

BREAKFAST   Time _____ Total Carb_____

      Serving Size   Food and Drinks

Grain
Vegetable
Protein
Fruit
Milk
Fat

SNACK   Time _____ Total Carb_____

LUNCH   Time _____ Total Carb_____

      Serving Size   Food and Drinks

Grain
Vegetable
Protein
Fruit
Milk
Fat

SNACK   Time _____ Total Carb_____

DINNER   Time _____ Total Carb_____

      Serving Size   Food and Drinks

Grain
Vegetable
Protein
Fruit
Milk
Fat

T O T A L S

VEGETABLES   FRUIT   NUTS   WHOLE GRAINS

FUN	EMOTIONS	MOOD	ILLNESS	STRESS

Energy Level   1   2   3   4   5   6   7   8   9   10

MOVEMENT

Time of Day   Comments

Walking _____ steps/minutes

Weights _____ lbs, _____ reps

Stretches _____ minutes

Laughter _____

Other _____   **Weight** _____

BLOOD GLUCOSE NUMBERS

Time	Breakfast Before	Breakfast After	Lunch Before	Lunch After	Dinner Before	Dinner After	Bedtime

MEDICATIONS

Time	Type

Carbohydrates

Complex (good) carbohydrates are in whole grains, fruits, vegetables, and beans, and give you vitamins, minerals, fiber, and antioxidants, so you are healthy! These carbohydrates are your body's best fuel. Simple (bad) carbohydrates are found in products with sugars and white flour such as soda, desserts, snacks, and juices. You can eat them, just don't eat much. They've lost their fiber, vitamins, and minerals.

Total Carbohydrate is listed on food labels:
　Sugars　(goal: only 20% of your total carbs daily)
　Fiber　(goal: 20–25 grams of fiber a day)

The outside aisles of grocery stores are where you find fiber-rich fruits, vegetables, and grains. You may have to go in an aisle or two to find the beans, which are full of fiber, too. Look for vibrant red, yellow, green, and orange in your fruit and vegetables. Fiber helps keep digestion healthy and may lower heart disease and cancer risk.

—Leslie Bonci, MPH, RD
American Dietetic Association Spokesperson

Date _____ Deep Breathing _____ Sleep _____

HOURS

Water ☐ ☐ ☐ ☐ ☐ ☐ ☐ ☐ Blood Pressure _____

F O O D

BREAKFAST

Time _____ Total Carb_____

	Serving Size	Food and Drinks
Grain		
Vegetable		
Protein		
Fruit		
Milk		
Fat		

SNACK

Time _____ Total Carb_____

LUNCH

Time _____ Total Carb_____

	Serving Size	Food and Drinks
Grain		
Vegetable		
Protein		
Fruit		
Milk		
Fat		

SNACK

Time _____ Total Carb_____

DINNER

Time _____ Total Carb_____

	Serving Size	Food and Drinks
Grain		
Vegetable		
Protein		
Fruit		
Milk		
Fat		

T O T A L S

VEGETABLES   FRUIT   NUTS   WHOLE GRAINS

Energy Level 1 2 3 4 5 6 7 8 9 10

MOVEMENT

Time of Day   Comments

Walking _____ steps/minutes

Weights _____ lbs, _____ reps

Stretches _____ minutes

Laughter _____

Other _____ **Weight** _____

BLOOD GLUCOSE NUMBERS							
	Breakfast		Lunch		Dinner		
Time	Before	After	Before	After	Before	After	Bedtime

MEDICATIONS	
Time	Type

Antioxidants

The body is a slow furnace burning the fats, carbohydrates, and protein that we eat. This process also produces carbon dioxide, water, and occasionally, free radicals. Free radicals bump into and damage cells and DNA and interfere with our natural cancer-fighting defenses. We have repair systems and natural antioxidants in the body, but we also need antioxidants in our food to fight the free radicals.

Fruits and vegetables give you a wonderful selection of antioxidants—it's nature's mix. We need at least 5 servings of fruits and vegetables each day, but the average person eats only 3 servings or LESS. The American Cancer Society recommends 9 or more servings daily. Hurry and catch up! Look for colorful vegetables to find foods rich in antioxidants.

—Phyllis Bowen, PhD
Associate Professor at University of Illinois

Date _____ Deep Breathing _____ Sleep _____
HOURS

Water ⊔ ⊔ ⊔ ⊔ ⊔ ⊔ ⊔ ⊔   Blood Pressure _____

F O O D

BREAKFAST   Time _____ Total Carb_____

      Serving Size   Food and Drinks

Grain
Vegetable
Protein
Fruit
Milk
Fat

SNACK   Time _____ Total Carb_____

LUNCH   Time _____ Total Carb_____

      Serving Size   Food and Drinks

Grain
Vegetable
Protein
Fruit
Milk
Fat

SNACK   Time _____ Total Carb_____

DINNER   Time _____ Total Carb_____

      Serving Size   Food and Drinks

Grain
Vegetable
Protein
Fruit
Milk
Fat

T O T A L S

VEGETABLES   FRUIT   NUTS   WHOLE GRAINS

FUN	EMOTIONS	MOOD	ILLNESS	STRESS

Energy Level   1   2   3   4   5   6   7   8   9   10

MOVEMENT

Time of Day   Comments

Walking _____ steps/minutes

Weights _____ lbs, _____ reps

Stretches _____ minutes

Laughter _____

Other _____   **Weight** _____

BLOOD GLUCOSE NUMBERS

Time	Breakfast		Lunch		Dinner		Bedtime
	Before	After	Before	After	Before	After	

MEDICATIONS

Time	Type

Aerobic Exercise

- Is rhythmic, steady activity involving most of your body.
- Works the heart and cardiovascular system, making them healthier.
- Encourages blood flow to the parts of the body that help us move and function.
- Can increase HDL (good) cholesterol.
- Can lower blood pressure (an average of 10 points). Some people can even go off blood pressure meds (fewer side effects and money saved).
- Makes the body sensitive to insulin, leading to good blood sugar levels.

The key is to move a little more and eat a little less!
- Do at least 20 minutes a day total—you can break it into 5- or 10-minute segments.
- Be able to carry on a normal conversation while you are exercising.
- The best time is the time that you will do it regularly.
- Exercise 5–7 days a week for weight loss and at least 3 times for weight maintenance.

—Cedric X. Bryant, PhD
VP, Product Management and Sports Medicine,
StairMaster Corporation

Date _____ Deep Breathing _____ Sleep _____
HOURS

Water ⊔ ⊔ ⊔ ⊔ ⊔ ⊔ ⊔ ⊔   Blood Pressure _____

F O O D

BREAKFAST   Time _____ Total Carb_____

    Serving Size   Food and Drinks

Grain
Vegetable
Protein
Fruit
Milk
Fat

_____

SNACK   Time _____ Total Carb_____

_____

LUNCH   Time _____ Total Carb_____

    Serving Size   Food and Drinks

Grain
Vegetable
Protein
Fruit
Milk
Fat

_____

SNACK   Time _____ Total Carb_____

_____

DINNER   Time _____ Total Carb_____

    Serving Size   Food and Drinks

Grain
Vegetable
Protein
Fruit
Milk
Fat

_____

T O T A L S

VEGETABLES   FRUIT   NUTS   WHOLE GRAINS

FUN	EMOTIONS	MOOD	ILLNESS	STRESS

Energy Level 1 2 3 4 5 6 7 8 9 10

MOVEMENT

Time of Day   Comments

Walking _____ steps/minutes

Weights _____ lbs, _____ reps

Stretches _____ minutes

Laughter _____

Other _____   **Weight** _____

BLOOD GLUCOSE NUMBERS

Time	Breakfast		Lunch		Dinner		Bedtime
	Before	After	Before	After	Before	After	

MEDICATIONS

Time	Type

Healthy Insight for the Day

GRAHAM

How to hard boil and shell an egg. Put the eggs in the bottom of a saucepan in cold water, and bring it to a boil. When it hits the boil, take the pan off the heat and put a lid on it. Let it sit for 15 minutes. You will have a perfect hard-boiled egg. To shell the egg, pour off the water and shake the eggs around in the pan. This movement breaks the shells and makes it easy to peel the eggs.

To peel a tomato, place it in boiling water for thirty seconds, and then transfer it to a bowl of iced water. This helps loosen the skin on the tomato and makes it easier to peel.

Date _____ Deep Breathing _____ Sleep _____
HOURS

Water ☐ ☐ ☐ ☐ ☐ ☐ ☐ ☐   Blood Pressure _____

F O O D

BREAKFAST   Time _____ Total Carb_____

	Serving Size	Food and Drinks
Grain		
Vegetable		
Protein		
Fruit		
Milk		
Fat		

SNACK   Time _____ Total Carb_____

LUNCH   Time _____ Total Carb_____

	Serving Size	Food and Drinks
Grain		
Vegetable		
Protein		
Fruit		
Milk		
Fat		

SNACK   Time _____ Total Carb_____

DINNER   Time _____ Total Carb_____

	Serving Size	Food and Drinks
Grain		
Vegetable		
Protein		
Fruit		
Milk		
Fat		

T O T A L S

VEGETABLES   FRUIT   NUTS   WHOLE GRAINS

Energy Level 1   2   3   4   5   6   7   8   9   10

MOVEMENT

Time of Day   Comments

Walking _____ steps/minutes

Weights _____ lbs, _____ reps

Stretches _____ minutes

Laughter _____

Other _____   **Weight** _____

	BLOOD GLUCOSE NUMBERS						
	Breakfast		Lunch		Dinner		
Time	Before	After	Before	After	Before	After	Bedtime

MEDICATIONS	
Time	Type

Biotechnology

Biotechnology is a step beyond cross-breeding plants. In cross-breeding, you select seeds from plants with the traits you want and sow them together, to try to get those traits in the next crop. Biotechnology removes a trait from a plant and puts it into another plant. Many foods today have been touched by biotechnology: corn, soybeans, and potatoes (25–75% of these crops). They are not labeled because they are not substantially different from traditional foods.

We've practiced biotechnology for 3,800 years since we first learned to ferment grapes into wine. Another ancient food is cheese, which was made with rennet. Now half of all cheese we buy has been made with an enzyme called chymesin.

A word of warning: If you are allergic to a food, say peanuts, you may also be allergic to a food that has received traits from peanuts through biotechnology. So, researchers are careful to avoid foods with allergenic properties.

—Felicia Busch, MPH, RD
American Dietetic Association Spokesperson

Date _____ Deep Breathing _____ Sleep _____
HOURS

Water 🥛 🥛 🥛 🥛 🥛 🥛 🥛 🥛   Blood Pressure _____

F O O D

BREAKFAST   Time _____ Total Carb_____

      Serving Size   Food and Drinks
Grain
Vegetable
Protein
Fruit
Milk
Fat

SNACK   Time _____ Total Carb_____

LUNCH   Time _____ Total Carb_____

      Serving Size   Food and Drinks
Grain
Vegetable
Protein
Fruit
Milk
Fat

SNACK   Time _____ Total Carb_____

DINNER   Time _____ Total Carb_____

      Serving Size   Food and Drinks
Grain
Vegetable
Protein
Fruit
Milk
Fat

TOTALS

VEGETABLES   FRUIT   NUTS   WHOLE GRAINS

FUN	EMOTIONS	MOOD	ILLNESS	STRESS

Energy Level 1 2 3 4 5 6 7 8 9 10

MOVEMENT

Time of Day   Comments

Walking _____ steps/minutes

Weights _____ lbs, _____ reps

Stretches _____ minutes

Laughter _____

Other _____ **Weight** _____

BLOCK GLUCOSE NUMBERS							
	Breakfast		Lunch		Dinner		
Time	Before	After	Before	After	Before	After	Bedtime

MEDICATIONS	
Time	Type

Strength Training

Strength training builds muscle tone, protects bones and joints, and burns calories. It makes you feel better by raising levels of endorphins and serotonin (feel-good hormones). Muscle burns calories even at rest—the larger the muscle, the more calories it guzzles.

As we age, we lose muscle unless we do something. Research shows 90-year-olds with walkers could walk on their own after 3 months of strength training. Hip fractures are common after age 65 if the muscles are too weak to protect the joint. Strength training is an investment in your future!

Muscles respond to resistance—be it a person, a jug of laundry soap, or a 2-lb bag of rice. You don't need expensive equipment. You can build muscles in 15–20 minutes 2–3 times a week— less than an hour a week! Find a fitness professional certified by the American College of Sports Medicine (ACSM), and get an exercise plan that is right for you.

—Cedric X. Bryant, PhD
VP, Product Management and Sports Medicine,
StairMaster Corporation

Date _____ Deep Breathing _____ Sleep _____

Water ▯ ▯ ▯ ▯ ▯ ▯ ▯ ▯   Blood Pressure _____

HOURS

F O O D

BREAKFAST
Time _____ Total Carb_____

	Serving Size	Food and Drinks
Grain		
Vegetable		
Protein		
Fruit		
Milk		
Fat		

SNACK
Time _____ Total Carb_____

LUNCH
Time _____ Total Carb_____

	Serving Size	Food and Drinks
Grain		
Vegetable		
Protein		
Fruit		
Milk		
Fat		

SNACK
Time _____ Total Carb_____

DINNER
Time _____ Total Carb_____

	Serving Size	Food and Drinks
Grain		
Vegetable		
Protein		
Fruit		
Milk		
Fat		

T O T A L S

VEGETABLES   FRUIT   NUTS   WHOLE GRAINS

FUN	EMOTIONS	MOOD	ILLNESS	STRESS

Energy Level 1 2 3 4 5 6 7 8 9 10

MOVEMENT

Time of Day   Comments

Walking _____ steps/minutes

Weights _____ lbs, _____ reps

Stretches _____ minutes

Laughter _____

Other _____ **Weight** _____

BLOOD GLUCOSE NUMBERS							
	Breakfast		Lunch		Dinner		
Time	Before	After	Before	After	Before	After	Bedtime

MEDICATIONS	
Time	Type

To Prevent Arthritis

Watch your weight. If you can lose just 10 pounds, you are less likely to get arthritis.

Using large-grip products puts less pressure on your joints.

If You Have Arthritis

- The earlier you go to see a rheumatologist, the better you will manage the disease.
- Hot compresses, baths, creams, and paraffin wax may relieve pain.
- Work with trained physical therapists who specialize in arthritis.
- Aspirin is good for arthritis and often a first therapy; check with your doctor.
- Some nightshade vegetables (eggplant, green peppers), chocolate, sugars, and milk products may make the disease worse in some individuals.

Don't be afraid of arthritis, instead, learn about it and take control. More information at www.arthritis.org

—Leigh Callahan, PhD
Arthritis Research Center, University of North Carolina

Date _____ Deep Breathing _____ Sleep _____
HOURS

Water ☐ ☐ ☐ ☐ ☐ ☐ ☐ ☐   Blood Pressure _____

F O O D

BREAKFAST   Time _____ Total Carb_____

  Serving Size   Food and Drinks

Grain
Vegetable
Protein
Fruit
Milk
Fat

SNACK   Time _____ Total Carb_____

LUNCH   Time _____ Total Carb_____

  Serving Size   Food and Drinks

Grain
Vegetable
Protein
Fruit
Milk
Fat

SNACK   Time _____ Total Carb_____

DINNER   Time _____ Total Carb_____

  Serving Size   Food and Drinks

Grain
Vegetable
Protein
Fruit
Milk
Fat

T O T A L S

VEGETABLES   FRUIT   NUTS   WHOLE GRAINS

FUN	EMOTIONS	MOOD	ILLNESS	STRESS

Energy Level   1   2   3   4   5   6   7   8   9   10

MOVEMENT

Time of Day   Comments

Walking _____ steps/minutes

Weights _____ lbs, _____ reps

Stretches _____ minutes

Laughter _____

Other _____   **Weight** _____

BLOOD GLUCOSE NUMBERS

Time	Breakfast		Lunch		Dinner		Bedtime
	Before	After	Before	After	Before	After	

MEDICATIONS

Time	Type

Insulin Resistance

You may have Insulin Resistance Syndrome (IRS) if you are overweight with an "apple" shape or a large stomach, high blood pressure, high triglycerides, low HDL cholesterol, and higher than normal blood sugar levels. You may make 2 to 4 times or more insulin to digest your food, but still cannot keep blood sugar normal. You need to lose some weight now. Why? IRS greatly increases your chances of getting cancer, heart disease, and diabetes.

1. Know your numbers (fasting blood sugar, triglycerides, total, and HDL cholesterol)
2. Look at your eating patterns and try to eat sensibly and enjoy.
3. Some exercise (30 minutes 5 times a week) is the key to weight loss and healing.
4. Look at the whole picture of your life, and see what to change first, one step at a time.
5. Starting to lose weight now prevents diabetes.

IRS gets worse as we get older and is compounded by our culture's sedentary ways.

—Wayne Calloway, MD
Professor of Medicine, George Washington University

Date _____ Deep Breathing _____ Sleep _____
HOURS

Water 🥛 🥛 🥛 🥛 🥛 🥛 🥛 🥛   Blood Pressure _____

F O O D

BREAKFAST   Time _____ Total Carb_____

Serving Size	Food and Drinks
Grain	
Vegetable	
Protein	
Fruit	
Milk	
Fat	

SNACK   Time _____ Total Carb_____

LUNCH   Time _____ Total Carb_____

Serving Size	Food and Drinks
Grain	
Vegetable	
Protein	
Fruit	
Milk	
Fat	

SNACK   Time _____ Total Carb_____

DINNER   Time _____ Total Carb_____

Serving Size	Food and Drinks
Grain	
Vegetable	
Protein	
Fruit	
Milk	
Fat	

T O T A L S

VEGETABLES   FRUIT   NUTS   WHOLE GRAINS

FUN	EMOTIONS	MOOD	ILLNESS	STRESS

Energy Level   1   2   3   4   5   6   7   8   9   10

MOVEMENT

Time of Day   Comments

Walking _____ steps/minutes

Weights _____ lbs, _____ reps

Stretches _____ minutes

Laughter _____

Other _____   Weight _____

BLOOD GLUCOSE NUMBERS								MEDICATIONS	
	Breakfast		Lunch		Dinner			Time	Type
Time	Before	After	Before	After	Before	After	Bedtime		

Healthy Latin Cooking Packed with Flavor

Latin cooking—or the cooking of any culture's food—doesn't have to depend on fat to make it taste good. Use spices and fresh herbs of the country to get the taste you want. (EthniMix, *Charting a Course to Wellness,* pages 476–478.)

The primary techniques to use in low-fat Latin cooking:

1. Sofrito is the key to flavorful Latin food. It is a combination of onions, garlic, sweet peppers, and vinegar.
2. Almost as important are spices and fresh herbs, such as cilantro.

You don't need to have fat to make it taste good.

—Thais Carreno, Owner
Fat Busters Cantina Service

GRAHAM

You can work wonders with a native cuisine. Changes can be made, health can be achieved, and food can be enjoyed. Hang on to the foods that define who you are, and refine them a bit so that you can live longer, healthier and happier!

Date _____ Deep Breathing _____ Sleep _____
HOURS

Water ☐ ☐ ☐ ☐ ☐ ☐ ☐ ☐   Blood Pressure _____

F O O D

BREAKFAST
Time _____ Total Carb_____

    Serving Size   Food and Drinks

Grain
Vegetable
Protein
Fruit
Milk
Fat

SNACK
Time _____ Total Carb_____

LUNCH
Time _____ Total Carb_____

    Serving Size   Food and Drinks

Grain
Vegetable
Protein
Fruit
Milk
Fat

SNACK
Time _____ Total Carb_____

DINNER
Time _____ Total Carb_____

    Serving Size   Food and Drinks

Grain
Vegetable
Protein
Fruit
Milk
Fat

TOTALS

VEGETABLES   FRUIT   NUTS   WHOLE GRAINS

FUN	EMOTIONS	MOOD	ILLNESS	STRESS

Energy Level   1   2   3   4   5   6   7   8   9   10

MOVEMENT

Time of Day   Comments

Walking _____ steps/minutes

Weights _____ lbs, _____ reps

Stretches _____ minutes

Laughter _____

Other _____   Weight _____

BLOOD GLUCOSE NUMBERS

Time	Breakfast		Lunch		Dinner		Bedtime
	Before	After	Before	After	Before	After	

MEDICATIONS

Time	Type

Cholesterol Fact

Fifty percent of Americans will have a stroke or a heart attack. The average LDL cholesterol of someone who has a heart attack is 150mg/dl. Those who exercise the most have the lowest heart attack rate and live longest. They also have the lowest LDL levels. Whatever form of exercise you like is the best choice, because you will stick with it. (Walking 2 miles or burning 200 calories a day is best.) Also, don't eat so much saturated fat (animal fat and tropical oils). Eat well-balanced meals in reasonable servings. Your goal is to have an LDL <100 if you have established coronary disease (angina, stroke, heart attack, bypass surgery, or angioplasty).

—William Castelli, MD
Medical Director, Framingham Heart Study

GRAHAM

When decreasing fat, let taste, aroma, color, and texture (TACT) be your guide to tasty dishes. Find out your own numbers like LDL. Ask to be referred to a dietitian to learn how to decrease saturated fat and improve your diet. Most people prepare the same 10 dishes over and over, so search for creativity. Enrich your life.

Date _____ Deep Breathing _____ Sleep _____

HOURS

Water ⬜ ⬜ ⬜ ⬜ ⬜ ⬜ ⬜ ⬜   Blood Pressure _____

F O O D

BREAKFAST
Time _____ Total Carb_____

        Serving Size   Food and Drinks

Grain
Vegetable
Protein
Fruit
Milk
Fat

SNACK
Time _____ Total Carb_____

LUNCH
Time _____ Total Carb_____

        Serving Size   Food and Drinks

Grain
Vegetable
Protein
Fruit
Milk
Fat

SNACK
Time _____ Total Carb_____

DINNER
Time _____ Total Carb_____

        Serving Size   Food and Drinks

Grain
Vegetable
Protein
Fruit
Milk
Fat

T O T A L S

VEGETABLES   FRUIT   NUTS   WHOLE GRAINS

| FUN | EMOTIONS | MOOD | ILLNESS | STRESS |

Energy Level 1 2 3 4 5 6 7 8 9 10

MOVEMENT

Time of Day   Comments

Walking _____ steps/minutes

Weights _____ lbs, _____ reps

Stretches _____ minutes

Laughter _____

Other _____   **Weight** _____

BLOOD GLUCOSE NUMBERS

Time	Breakfast		Lunch		Dinner		Bedtime
	Before	After	Before	After	Before	After	

MEDICATIONS

Time	Type

Nutrition and Diabetes

Symptoms when blood sugar (glucose) is not getting into the cells:

- Tired
- Irritable
- Blurred vision
- Can't think clearly

Myth: Avoid fruit when you have diabetes. **Fact:** Fruit fits in a diabetic meal plan. Spread your fruit servings over the day to prevent a spike in blood glucose levels. Three servings of fruit daily should be fine for most people.

Myth: You can't eat certain foods when you have diabetes. **Fact:** There are no foods to avoid. There are some that are better choices, but all foods can fit in your meal plan. If you focus on a wide variety of foods, keep your weight under control, stay active, and eat a diet that limits fat and focuses on "good" carbohydrates, your blood sugar will be where it should be, and you'll feel fine.

—**Karen A. Chalmers, MD, RD, CDE**
Director of Nutrition Services, Joslin Diabetes Center

Date _____ Deep Breathing _____ Sleep _____
HOURS

Water ☐ ☐ ☐ ☐ ☐ ☐ ☐ ☐   Blood Pressure _____

F O O D

BREAKFAST   Time _____ Total Carb_____

      Serving Size   Food and Drinks

Grain
Vegetable
Protein
Fruit
Milk
Fat

SNACK   Time _____ Total Carb_____

LUNCH   Time _____ Total Carb_____

      Serving Size   Food and Drinks

Grain
Vegetable
Protein
Fruit
Milk
Fat

SNACK   Time _____ Total Carb_____

DINNER   Time _____ Total Carb_____

      Serving Size   Food and Drinks

Grain
Vegetable
Protein
Fruit
Milk
Fat

T O T A L S

VEGETABLES   FRUIT   NUTS   WHOLE GRAINS

FUN	EMOTIONS	MOOD	ILLNESS	STRESS

Energy Level 1 2 3 4 5 6 7 8 9 10

MOVEMENT

Time of Day   Comments

Walking _____ steps/minutes

Weights _____ lbs, _____ reps

Stretches _____ minutes

Laughter _____

Other _____   **Weight** _____

BLOOD GLUCOSE NUMBERS

Time	Breakfast		Lunch		Dinner		Bedtime
	Before	After	Before	After	Before	After	

MEDICATIONS

Time	Type

Caffeine

A moderate coffee drinker has 2 1/2 cups each day or about 200–300 mg of caffeine. The amount of caffeine depends on preparation methods and brands:

Brewed coffee (8 oz)	85 mg
Instant coffee (8 oz)	75 mg
Brewed tea (8 oz)	40 mg
Instant tea (8 oz)	28 mg
Iced tea (8 oz)	25 mg
Cola-type soda (8 oz)	24 mg
Dark chocolate (1 oz)	20 mg

Some medications contain caffeine. Ask your doctor or pharmacist if you are concerned. When trying a new beverage (like herbal coffee): Prepare it just as you have coffee in the past. Try three times, and on the third day, you will like it better. Don't expect it to taste the same as the beverage you are trying to replace, and try to like it for what it is.

—Stephen Cherniske, MS
Author, *Caffeine Blues*

Date _____ Deep Breathing _____ Sleep _____
HOURS

Water ☐ ☐ ☐ ☐ ☐ ☐ ☐ ☐   Blood Pressure _____

F O O D

BREAKFAST   Time _____ Total Carb_____

Serving Size   Food and Drinks

Grain
Vegetable
Protein
Fruit
Milk
Fat

SNACK   Time _____ Total Carb_____

LUNCH   Time _____ Total Carb_____

Serving Size   Food and Drinks

Grain
Vegetable
Protein
Fruit
Milk
Fat

SNACK   Time _____ Total Carb_____

DINNER   Time _____ Total Carb_____

Serving Size   Food and Drinks

Grain
Vegetable
Protein
Fruit
Milk
Fat

TOTALS

VEGETABLES   FRUIT   NUTS   WHOLE GRAINS

FUN	EMOTIONS	MOOD	ILLNESS	STRESS

Energy Level 1 2 3 4 5 6 7 8 9 10

MOVEMENT

Time of Day   Comments

Walking _____ steps/minutes

Weights _____ lbs, _____ reps

Stretches _____ minutes

Laughter _____

Other _____   **Weight** _____

BLOOD GLUCOSE NUMBERS

Time	Breakfast		Lunch		Dinner		Bedtime
	Before	After	Before	After	Before	After	

MEDICATIONS

Time	Type

Calories

Calories measure how much fuel you put in your body.

Choose a reasonable weight for yourself and multiply by 10 to get the calories you need just to lie down all day (resting metabolic rate). Example: 140 pounds × 10 = 1,400 calories

Add half that number for moving around: 1,400 + 700 = 2,100 calories

Add 300–400 calories if you are high-energy or exercise regularly. Don't add anything if you just sit all day. To lose weight, subtract 20% of your daily calorie needs.

2,100 × 0.20 = 420 calories; 2100 − 420 = 1,680 calories for weight loss

To Cut Calories

- Eat breakfast and lunch so you don't overeat later.
- Eat only when you are truly hungry.
- Watch serving sizes, so you don't eat too much.

Exercise burns calories, and it also relieves stress, and makes you feel good. Strength training is important, because the more muscle you have, the more calories you burn even at rest. Just start moving, even the smallest amounts of exercise help you feel better.

—Nancy Clark, MS, RD
Author, *Sports Nutrition Guidebook*

Date _____ Deep Breathing _____ Sleep _____
HOURS

Water ⊔ ⊔ ⊔ ⊔ ⊔ ⊔ ⊔ ⊔   Blood Pressure _____

F O O D

BREAKFAST   Time _____ Total Carb_____

	Serving Size	Food and Drinks
Grain		
Vegetable		
Protein		
Fruit		
Milk		
Fat		

SNACK   Time _____ Total Carb_____

LUNCH   Time _____ Total Carb_____

	Serving Size	Food and Drinks
Grain		
Vegetable		
Protein		
Fruit		
Milk		
Fat		

SNACK   Time _____ Total Carb_____

DINNER   Time _____ Total Carb_____

	Serving Size	Food and Drinks
Grain		
Vegetable		
Protein		
Fruit		
Milk		
Fat		

T O T A L S

VEGETABLES   FRUIT   NUTS   WHOLE GRAINS

FUN	EMOTIONS	MOOD	ILLNESS	STRESS

Energy Level 1 2 3 4 5 6 7 8 9 10

MOVEMENT

Time of Day   Comments

Walking _____ steps/minutes

Weights _____ lbs, _____ reps

Stretches _____ minutes

Laughter _____

Other _____ **Weight** _____

BLOOD GLUCOSE NUMBERS

Time	Breakfast		Lunch		Dinner		Bedtime
	Before	After	Before	After	Before	After	

MEDICATIONS

Time	Type

School Food Programs

Our children are flunking eating. School children eat less than 1 serving of fruit a day and few vegetables or whole grains. Poor eating habits and inactivity are causing overweight and obesity. The number of overweight children and teens has doubled in 30 years. Children who eat a school lunch eat more milk, fruits, and vegetables than children who bring their lunches from home. Kids who eat the school breakfast program have improved test scores and are healthier and better behaved.

You can help change how children eat! Encourage better meals and daily physical education at school. Be sure schools are serving healthy choices in the cafeteria and vending machines. Make sure the school schedules meals when children are hungry—not at 10 AM or 2 PM—and provides enough time for them to enjoy their meals. Teach students and parents about healthy food choices and get them involved.

—**Martha Conklin, PhD, RD**
Co-Author, *Managing Child Nutrition Programs*

Date _____ Deep Breathing _____ Sleep _____

Water ⬜ ⬜ ⬜ ⬜ ⬜ ⬜ ⬜ ⬜   Blood Pressure _____ HOURS

F O O D

BREAKFAST   Time _____ Total Carb_____

	Serving Size	Food and Drinks
Grain		
Vegetable		
Protein		
Fruit		
Milk		
Fat		

SNACK   Time _____ Total Carb_____

LUNCH   Time _____ Total Carb_____

	Serving Size	Food and Drinks
Grain		
Vegetable		
Protein		
Fruit		
Milk		
Fat		

SNACK   Time _____ Total Carb_____

DINNER   Time _____ Total Carb_____

	Serving Size	Food and Drinks
Grain		
Vegetable		
Protein		
Fruit		
Milk		
Fat		

T O T A L S

VEGETABLES   FRUIT   NUTS   WHOLE GRAINS

Energy Level 1 2 3 4 5 6 7 8 9 10

MOVEMENT

Time of Day   Comments

Walking _____ steps/minutes

Weights _____ lbs, _____ reps

Stretches _____ minutes

Laughter _____

Other _____   Weight _____

BLOOD GLUCOSE NUMBERS

| Time | Breakfast | | Lunch | | Dinner | | Bedtime |
	Before	After	Before	After	Before	After	

MEDICATIONS

Time	Type

Omega-3 Fats

The body needs polyunsaturated fats—especially omega-3 fats—to be healthy, so you need to eat foods containing them, such as fish, olive oil, and flaxseed. Many processed foods, even some vegetable oils, have lots of omega-6 fats, but very few omega-3s. You need these healthy fats in balanced amounts, so try to get more omega-3s. Use olive or canola oil, and grind flaxseeds to sprinkle on cereal and baked goods. Omega-3s keep fat metabolism in balance and cholesterol levels healthy, reduce the tendency for blood to clot, and steady the heart's rhythm.

Fish get omega-3 fats from eating smaller fish that eat cold-water plants. Fish in your meals 1 or 2 times a week can replace meats with saturated fat. The colder the water the higher the health value of fish, like salmon and mackerel. Farm fish have less omega-3s than wild fish, but they also have less mercury than ocean fish, such as tuna. Mercury is bad for you. Fresh fish is a better choice than fish oil supplements.

—Stephen Cunnane, PhD
Researcher and Professor, University of Toronto

Date _____ Deep Breathing _____ Sleep _____
HOURS

Water 🥛 🥛 🥛 🥛 🥛 🥛 🥛 🥛   Blood Pressure _____

F O O D

BREAKFAST   Time _____ Total Carb_____

	Serving Size	Food and Drinks
Grain		
Vegetable		
Protein		
Fruit		
Milk		
Fat		

SNACK   Time _____ Total Carb_____

LUNCH   Time _____ Total Carb_____

	Serving Size	Food and Drinks
Grain		
Vegetable		
Protein		
Fruit		
Milk		
Fat		

SNACK   Time _____ Total Carb_____

DINNER   Time _____ Total Carb_____

	Serving Size	Food and Drinks
Grain		
Vegetable		
Protein		
Fruit		
Milk		
Fat		

T O T A L S

VEGETABLES   FRUIT   NUTS   WHOLE GRAINS

FUN	EMOTIONS	MOOD	ILLNESS	STRESS

Energy Level 1 2 3 4 5 6 7 8 9 10

MOVEMENT

Time of Day   Comments

Walking _____ steps/minutes

Weights _____ lbs, _____ reps

Stretches _____ minutes

Laughter _____

Other _____   **Weight** _____

BLOOD GLUCOSE NUMBERS

Time	Breakfast		Lunch		Dinner		Bedtime
	Before	After	Before	After	Before	After	

MEDICATIONS

Time	Type

Osteoporosis

Osteoporosis is a loss of calcium from bones, resulting in a fracture. After age 25, women gradually lose some bone mass until menopause, when the loss may speed up. This disease can be painful. Men may develop osteoporosis 10 years later than women.

We all need to get calcium. The recommended amount is: 1,500 mg calcium a day for postmenopausal women and 1200 mg for most others. Foods with calcium are:

Skim milk	300 mg per cup
Bok Choy	160 mg per cup
Broccoli	100 mg per cup
Spinach and Collard Greens	100–120 mg per cup

Evaporated milk has twice the amount of calcium as regular milk. Yogurt, cheese, and calcium-fortified foods like orange juice are also great sources.

—Chad Deal, MD
Head, Center for Osteoporosis, The Cleveland Clinic Foundation

Date _____ Deep Breathing _____ Sleep _____
HOURS

Water ☐ ☐ ☐ ☐ ☐ ☐ ☐ ☐ Blood Pressure _____

F O O D

BREAKFAST Time _____ Total Carb_____

Serving Size   Food and Drinks

Grain
Vegetable
Protein
Fruit
Milk
Fat

SNACK Time _____ Total Carb_____

LUNCH Time _____ Total Carb_____

Serving Size   Food and Drinks

Grain
Vegetable
Protein
Fruit
Milk
Fat

SNACK Time _____ Total Carb_____

DINNER Time _____ Total Carb_____

Serving Size   Food and Drinks

Grain
Vegetable
Protein
Fruit
Milk
Fat

TOTALS

VEGETABLES   FRUIT   NUTS   WHOLE GRAINS

FUN	EMOTIONS	MOOD	ILLNESS	STRESS

Energy Level 1 2 3 4 5 6 7 8 9 10

MOVEMENT

Time of Day   Comments

Walking _____ steps/minutes

Weights _____ lbs, _____ reps

Stretches _____ minutes

Laughter _____

Other _____   **Weight** _____

BLOOD GLUCOSE NUMBERS

Time	Breakfast		Lunch		Dinner		Bedtime
	Before	After	Before	After	Before	After	

MEDICATIONS

Time	Type

Osteoporosis

The best exercise for strong bones is weight-bearing. Swimming doesn't do it. You need a heel-strike exercise, which means putting your foot to the ground. A simple walking program, 30–40 minutes 4 times a week, saves your bones. Walking also helps prevent falls—you are a lot less likely to fall if you have been a lifelong exerciser.

Smoking and alcohol affect bone health. A woman who is a lifelong smoker has double the risk for fractures during her life. Smoking tends to make estrogen less effective. One of the most common causes of osteoporosis in men is too much alcohol.

To prevent osteoporosis: Encourage kids to get enough calcium and exercise as bones are developing. Adults need to do weight-bearing exercise and eat enough calcium. Stop smoking. Drink no more than one or two alcoholic drinks a day.

—Chad Deal, MD
Head, Center for Osteoporosis, The Cleveland Clinic
Foundation

Date _____ Deep Breathing _____ Sleep _____
HOURS

Water ▯ ▯ ▯ ▯ ▯ ▯ ▯ ▯   Blood Pressure _____

F O O D

BREAKFAST   Time _____ Total Carb_____

      Serving Size   Food and Drinks

Grain
Vegetable
Protein
Fruit
Milk
Fat

SNACK   Time _____ Total Carb_____

LUNCH   Time _____ Total Carb_____

      Serving Size   Food and Drinks

Grain
Vegetable
Protein
Fruit
Milk
Fat

SNACK   Time _____ Total Carb_____

DINNER   Time _____ Total Carb_____

      Serving Size   Food and Drinks

Grain
Vegetable
Protein
Fruit
Milk
Fat

TOTALS

VEGETABLES   FRUIT   NUTS   WHOLE GRAINS

FUN	EMOTIONS	MOOD	ILLNESS	STRESS

Energy Level 1 2 3 4 5 6 7 8 9 10

MOVEMENT

Time of Day   Comments

Walking _____ steps/minutes

Weights _____ lbs, _____ reps

Stretches _____ minutes

Laughter _____

Other _____ **Weight** _____

BLOOD GLUCOSE NUMBERS

Time	Breakfast		Lunch		Dinner		Bedtime
	Before	After	Before	After	Before	After	

MEDICATIONS

Time	Type

Hypertension

One in four adults (50 million people) has high blood pressure. Hypertension is blood pressure above 130/80. The top number (systolic) is pressure on arteries as the heart beats. The bottom number (diastolic) is pressure on arteries between beats. Think of the pressure on a water hose. Hypertension causes strokes, heart attacks, and kidney failure. Do you have hypertension? Often there are no symptoms until the heart attack or stroke. It is a "silent killer." You can treat it with weight loss, eating well, and exercise.

Some people are sensitive to salt. Most people eat about 4 grams a day (1 tsp salt). You can half it (2–2.5 grams) to see if this helps. Canned and processed foods have a lot of sodium, but fresh fruits and vegetables don't. You may also want to eat foods, such as bananas, with potassium, because it balances sodium and can help lower blood pressure.

—**Janice Douglas, MD**
Chief, Division of Hypertension, Case Western
Reserve University

Date _____ Deep Breathing _____ Sleep _____
HOURS

Water ☐ ☐ ☐ ☐ ☐ ☐ ☐ ☐   Blood Pressure _____

F O O D

BREAKFAST   Time _____ Total Carb_____

	Serving Size	Food and Drinks
Grain		
Vegetable		
Protein		
Fruit		
Milk		
Fat		

SNACK   Time _____ Total Carb_____

LUNCH   Time _____ Total Carb_____

	Serving Size	Food and Drinks
Grain		
Vegetable		
Protein		
Fruit		
Milk		
Fat		

SNACK   Time _____ Total Carb_____

DINNER   Time _____ Total Carb_____

	Serving Size	Food and Drinks
Grain		
Vegetable		
Protein		
Fruit		
Milk		
Fat		

T O T A L S

VEGETABLES   FRUIT   NUTS   WHOLE GRAINS

| FUN | EMOTIONS | MOOD | ILLNESS | STRESS |

Energy Level 1 2 3 4 5 6 7 8 9 10

MOVEMENT

Time of Day   Comments

Walking _____ steps/minutes

Weights _____ lbs, _____ reps

Stretches _____ minutes

Laughter _____

Other _____   **Weight** _____

BLOOD GLUCOSE NUMBERS							
	Breakfast		Lunch		Dinner		
Time	Before	After	Before	After	Before	After	Bedtime

MEDICATIONS	
Time	Type

Heart Disease—You Can Beat It

Heart disease affects 50% of us, and because we are an aging society, the rates will climb. Risk of heart disease, even in a healthy person, is much greater than other diseases. To reduce your risk of heart disease:

- Stop smoking.
- Lose weight if you need to.
- Lower high blood pressure. Use diet, exercise, and medication.
- Diabetes damages your heart and blood vessels unless it is well managed.
- Cut your heart risk in half with regular exercise. Walk 30 minutes a day most days of the week.
- Know your cholesterol level: total cholesterol, HDL, LDL and triglycerides. To lower cholesterol—eat better, exercise, and take medication if you need it.
- Aspirin is key—Men over 45 and women over 55 who take 1 baby aspirin or 1/2 regular aspirin a day reduce heart disease risk by 25%.

—Barry Effron, MD
Associate Chief of Cardiology, University Hospitals of Cleveland

Date _____ Deep Breathing _____ Sleep _____
HOURS

Water ☐ ☐ ☐ ☐ ☐ ☐ ☐ ☐ Blood Pressure _____

F O O D

BREAKFAST
Time _____ Total Carb _____

Serving Size	Food and Drinks
Grain	
Vegetable	
Protein	
Fruit	
Milk	
Fat	

SNACK
Time _____ Total Carb _____

LUNCH
Time _____ Total Carb _____

Serving Size	Food and Drinks
Grain	
Vegetable	
Protein	
Fruit	
Milk	
Fat	

SNACK
Time _____ Total Carb _____

DINNER
Time _____ Total Carb _____

Serving Size	Food and Drinks
Grain	
Vegetable	
Protein	
Fruit	
Milk	
Fat	

TOTALS

VEGETABLES   FRUIT   NUTS   WHOLE GRAINS

FUN	EMOTIONS	MOOD	ILLNESS	STRESS

Energy Level   1   2   3   4   5   6   7   8   9   10

MOVEMENT

Time of Day   Comments

Walking _____ steps/minutes

Weights _____ lbs, _____ reps

Stretches _____ minutes

Laughter _____

Other _____   **Weight** _____

BLOOD GLUCOSE NUMBERS

Time	Breakfast		Lunch		Dinner		Bedtime
	Before	After	Before	After	Before	After	

MEDICATIONS

Time	Type

Drinking Red Wine

The French have very low rates of heart disease, so researchers study them. Drinking red wine may be a key. The French diet is high in saturated fats; they smoke a lot and have high cholesterol levels, but they have only 1/3 the number of heart attacks that the United States has. Wine and de-alcoholized wines have antioxidants that protect hearts. Fermentation increases this protection. You get additional protection from alcohol that you don't get from de-alcoholized wine.

Drinking a moderate amount of alcohol is good, and abuse of alcohol is bad. One glass of wine a day with a meal can give you health benefits. You don't need more. A person with a family history of alcohol abuse should not drink, even for health purposes. One beer has the same benefit as a glass of wine. The French also eat lots of olive oil and vegetables and walk more than we do, too. Discuss drinking alcohol and other lifestyle changes with your physician before starting, especially when you are taking medication.

—**Curt Ellison, MD**
Chief of Preventive Medicine, Boston University

Date _____ Deep Breathing _____ Sleep _____
HOURS

Water ▢ ▢ ▢ ▢ ▢ ▢ ▢ ▢   Blood Pressure _____

F O O D

BREAKFAST   Time _____ Total Carb_____

      Serving Size   Food and Drinks

Grain
Vegetable
Protein
Fruit
Milk
Fat

SNACK   Time _____ Total Carb_____

LUNCH   Time _____ Total Carb_____

      Serving Size   Food and Drinks

Grain
Vegetable
Protein
Fruit
Milk
Fat

SNACK   Time _____ Total Carb_____

DINNER   Time _____ Total Carb_____

      Serving Size   Food and Drinks

Grain
Vegetable
Protein
Fruit
Milk
Fat

T O T A L S

VEGETABLES   FRUIT   NUTS   WHOLE GRAINS

Energy Level 1 2 3 4 5 6 7 8 9 10

MOVEMENT

Time of Day   Comments

Walking _____ steps/minutes

Weights _____ lbs, _____ reps

Stretches _____ minutes

Laughter _____

Other _____   **Weight** _____

	BLOOD GLUCOSE NUMBERS							MEDICATIONS	
	Breakfast		Lunch		Dinner			Time	Type
Time	Before	After	Before	After	Before	After	Bedtime		

Farmers and Food

Farmers' Markets: Get to know the people who grow your food—support them as they support you. Farmers can eliminate the middleman by selling their own crops, and you are helping them make a living when you buy at a farmers' market. The foods are fresh, great tasting, and in season. Locally grown in-season food is good for your family. You can help farmers save farmland by buying food from them.

Community Supported Agriculture (CSA): People in the community buy "shares" in the farm, which supplies capital for the farmers. As the produce is harvested, the shareholders come by to pick up their weekly supply of fresh, locally grown fruits, vegetables, herbs, and flowers. It works well for all concerned! If you're interested in learning more, call the Biodynamic Farming and Gardening Association in Pennsylvania. They keep a national registry of CSA farms and can tell you about one in your area. For general information on CSAs, write: CSA West, c/o University of California, P.O. Box 363, Davis, CA 95617 or on the Web go to www.nal.usda.gov/afsic/csa.

—**Gail Feenstra, MEd, EdD**
Food Systems Analyst, University of California, Davis

Date _____ Deep Breathing _____ Sleep _____
                                                                    HOURS

Water ▢ ▢ ▢ ▢ ▢ ▢ ▢ ▢   Blood Pressure _____

F O O D

BREAKFAST   Time _____ Total Carb_____

     Serving Size   Food and Drinks
Grain
Vegetable
Protein
Fruit
Milk
Fat

SNACK   Time _____ Total Carb_____

LUNCH   Time _____ Total Carb_____

     Serving Size   Food and Drinks
Grain
Vegetable
Protein
Fruit
Milk
Fat

SNACK   Time _____ Total Carb_____

DINNER   Time _____ Total Carb_____

     Serving Size   Food and Drinks
Grain
Vegetable
Protein
Fruit
Milk
Fat

TOTALS

VEGETABLES   FRUIT   NUTS   WHOLE GRAINS

FUN	EMOTIONS	MOOD	ILLNESS	STRESS

Energy Level   1   2   3   4   5   6   7   8   9   10

MOVEMENT

Time of Day   Comments

Walking _____ steps/minutes

Weights _____ lbs, _____ reps

Stretches _____ minutes

Laughter _____

Other _____   **Weight** _____

BLOOD GLUCOSE NUMBERS

Time	Breakfast		Lunch		Dinner		Bedtime
	Before	After	Before	After	Before	After	

MEDICATIONS

Time	Type

Breakfast

Research shows breakfast is a key to a healthier day. Breakfast feeds our bodies and our minds. Balanced breakfasts can raise our energy level and performance. Breakfast with a good balance of carbohydrate, protein, and fat sustains you until lunch and beyond.

Children who eat breakfast have a better attention span, think better, get to class on time, have fewer sick days, and fewer visits to the nurse. It's worth getting up earlier to fix a good breakfast.

- Increase calcium with fruit smoothies and cereal with milk.
- Increase fiber (20–35 grams a day) with whole grain cereals and breads and fruit.
- Increase fresh fruit, which is quick nutrition.
- Flaxseed, ground, can be added to recipes and sprinkled on cereals.
- Watch serving sizes to control calories.
- If you skip breakfast, you can't catch up, so start with nutritious foods.

—Cecilia Fileti, MS, RD, FADA
President, C.P. Fileti Associates, Inc.

Date _____ Deep Breathing _____ Sleep _____
HOURS

Water ☐ ☐ ☐ ☐ ☐ ☐ ☐ ☐ Blood Pressure _____

F O O D

BREAKFAST   Time _____ Total Carb_____

	Serving Size	Food and Drinks
Grain		
Vegetable		
Protein		
Fruit		
Milk		
Fat		

SNACK   Time _____ Total Carb_____

LUNCH   Time _____ Total Carb_____

	Serving Size	Food and Drinks
Grain		
Vegetable		
Protein		
Fruit		
Milk		
Fat		

SNACK   Time _____ Total Carb_____

DINNER   Time _____ Total Carb_____

	Serving Size	Food and Drinks
Grain		
Vegetable		
Protein		
Fruit		
Milk		
Fat		

TOTALS

VEGETABLES   FRUIT   NUTS   WHOLE GRAINS

FUN	EMOTIONS	MOOD	ILLNESS	STRESS

Energy Level 1 2 3 4 5 6 7 8 9 10

MOVEMENT

Time of Day   Comments

Walking _____ steps/minutes

Weights _____ lbs, _____ reps

Stretches _____ minutes

Laughter _____

Other _____

Weight _____

BLOOD GLUCOSE NUMBERS

Time	Breakfast		Lunch		Dinner		Bedtime
	Before	After	Before	After	Before	After	

MEDICATIONS

Time	Type

Self-Centered Dieting

Self-centered dieting is being preoccupied with your weight, your looks, and how you feel, which interferes with living your life. Self-centered dieting is unhealthy and often leads to failure. Well-being gives meaning to life. It is feeling good about yourself and your relationship with your world. Well-being makes it possible to love other people, to get on with living, and to reach out and help others. Then progress with weight control is likely. Successful weight control depends on moving your goal away from just weight loss to the meaning of your life and how you can help others.

Try the **100/100 plan** to reach a healthy weight: Cut 100 calories a day from your diet and burn 100 calories a day with a small amount of exercise such as walking 20 minutes. When you're upset and think about food, move your focus: call a friend, walk around the block, take a bath or shower, read a good book, or meditate.

—Dr. John Foreyt, PhD
Director, Behavioral Medicine Research,
Baylor School of Medicine

Date _____ Deep Breathing _____ Sleep _____
HOURS

Water ▯ ▯ ▯ ▯ ▯ ▯ ▯ ▯   Blood Pressure _____

F O O D

BREAKFAST
Time _____ Total Carb _____

	Serving Size	Food and Drinks
Grain		
Vegetable		
Protein		
Fruit		
Milk		
Fat		

SNACK
Time _____ Total Carb _____

LUNCH
Time _____ Total Carb _____

	Serving Size	Food and Drinks
Grain		
Vegetable		
Protein		
Fruit		
Milk		
Fat		

SNACK
Time _____ Total Carb _____

DINNER
Time _____ Total Carb _____

	Serving Size	Food and Drinks
Grain		
Vegetable		
Protein		
Fruit		
Milk		
Fat		

TOTALS

VEGETABLES   FRUIT   NUTS   WHOLE GRAINS

FUN	EMOTIONS	MOOD	ILLNESS	STRESS

Energy Level 1 2 3 4 5 6 7 8 9 10

MOVEMENT

Time of Day   Comments

Walking _____ steps/minutes

Weights _____ lbs, _____ reps

Stretches _____ minutes

Laughter _____

Other _____   **Weight** _____

BLOOD GLUCOSE NUMBERS

Time	Breakfast		Lunch		Dinner		Bedtime
	Before	After	Before	After	Before	After	

MEDICATIONS

Time	Type

Refined vs. Complex Carbohydrates

When foods are highly processed, a lot of healthful properties get removed, which is why they aren't so good for you. Unprocessed foods in their natural state have more vitamins, minerals, and nutrition. They are premium fuel. For example, fresh fruits are a better choice than juice, because fruit just has natural sugars (none added), and you get the benefit of fiber. And it hasn't sat on a shelf in a bottle or carton for several months or years. Add foods with fiber to your diet gradually so your body can adapt to it.

- Choose foods you enjoy, but watch the amount that you eat.
- Become more physically active.
- Make small changes, such as adding a fruit or vegetable to lunch and dinner today.

The healthiest choices for everyone are foods that are less processed and naturally contain more vitamins, minerals, and phytochemicals.

—Marion Franz, RD, MS
Director of Nutrition, International Diabetes Center, Minneapolis

Date _____ Deep Breathing _____ Sleep _____
HOURS

Water 🥛 🥛 🥛 🥛 🥛 🥛 🥛 🥛   Blood Pressure _____

F O O D

BREAKFAST   Time _____   Total Carb_____

     Serving Size   Food and Drinks

Grain
Vegetable
Protein
Fruit
Milk
Fat

SNACK   Time _____   Total Carb_____

LUNCH   Time _____   Total Carb_____

     Serving Size   Food and Drinks

Grain
Vegetable
Protein
Fruit
Milk
Fat

SNACK   Time _____   Total Carb_____

DINNER   Time _____   Total Carb_____

     Serving Size   Food and Drinks

Grain
Vegetable
Protein
Fruit
Milk
Fat

T O T A L S

VEGETABLES   FRUIT   NUTS   WHOLE GRAINS

Energy Level 1 2 3 4 5 6 7 8 9 10

MOVEMENT

Time of Day   Comments

Walking _____ steps/minutes

Weights _____ lbs, _____ reps

Stretches _____ minutes

Laughter _____

Other _____   **Weight** _____

BLOOD GLUCOSE NUMBERS							
	Breakfast		Lunch		Dinner		
Time	Before	After	Before	After	Before	After	Bedtime

MEDICATIONS	
Time	Type

Graham's Unique Techniques

- Canned beans are great for convenience, but they're high in sodium, so rinse first.
- Never put a knife through the dishwasher if you want to keep an edge on it.
- Graham's homemade vegetable stock recipe: 5 cups of water, parsley, carrot, leek, black peppercorns, turnip, onion chopped and sauteed with ginger and a touch of oil. Simmer thirty minutes and strain. Broth can be frozen.
- Roll a lemon on the countertop before you squeeze it to get the most juice extracted.

An appropriate serving of uncooked pasta is a 2-oz portion. Put cooked pasta in a colander standing in a bowl of steaming water. This will keep the pasta warm while you finish preparing the dish.

Date _____ Deep Breathing _____ Sleep _____
HOURS

Water ⬜ ⬜ ⬜ ⬜ ⬜ ⬜ ⬜ ⬜   Blood Pressure _____

F O O D

BREAKFAST   Time _____ Total Carb_____

       Serving Size   Food and Drinks

Grain
Vegetable
Protein
Fruit
Milk
Fat

SNACK   Time _____ Total Carb_____

LUNCH   Time _____ Total Carb_____

       Serving Size   Food and Drinks

Grain
Vegetable
Protein
Fruit
Milk
Fat

SNACK   Time _____ Total Carb_____

DINNER   Time _____ Total Carb_____

       Serving Size   Food and Drinks

Grain
Vegetable
Protein
Fruit
Milk
Fat

T O T A L S

VEGETABLES   FRUIT   NUTS   WHOLE GRAINS

Energy Level 1   2   3   4   5   6   7   8   9   10

MOVEMENT

Time of Day   Comments

Walking _____ steps/minutes

Weights _____ lbs, _____ reps

Stretches _____ minutes

Laughter _____

Other _____   **Weight** _____

BLOOD GLUCOSE NUMBERS

| Time | Breakfast | | Lunch | | Dinner | | Bedtime |
	Before	After	Before	After	Before	After	

MEDICATIONS

Time	Type

Diabetes Facts

There are 18 million Americans with diabetes, but only half know that they have it.

By keeping weight down in many cases, type 2 diabetes can be prevented—and if it develops, healthy weight helps control it. When a person loses 10–20 pounds, blood glucose levels often drop to normal.

Type 1 diabetes: More likely in young people; the pancreas makes no insulin, so they must take insulin injections. Type 2 diabetes: Comes on with weight, lack of activity, and aging; people may be able to manage it with lifestyle changes, but eventually the pancreas wears out and pills or insulin are necessary to keep blood glucose levels normal.

You want to keep your blood glucose near normal to avoid diabetic complications. Research shows that this truly works, so your efforts to manage your diabetes will be repaid with wellness.

—**Marion Franz, RD, MS**
Director of Nutrition, International Diabetes Center,
Minneapolis
www.idcdiabetes.org

Date _____ Deep Breathing _____ Sleep _____
HOURS

Water ⬜ ⬜ ⬜ ⬜ ⬜ ⬜ ⬜ ⬜   Blood Pressure _____

F O O D

BREAKFAST   Time _____ Total Carb_____

Serving Size	Food and Drinks
Grain	
Vegetable	
Protein	
Fruit	
Milk	
Fat	

SNACK   Time _____ Total Carb_____

LUNCH   Time _____ Total Carb_____

Serving Size	Food and Drinks
Grain	
Vegetable	
Protein	
Fruit	
Milk	
Fat	

SNACK   Time _____ Total Carb_____

DINNER   Time _____ Total Carb_____

Serving Size	Food and Drinks
Grain	
Vegetable	
Protein	
Fruit	
Milk	
Fat	

TOTALS

VEGETABLES   FRUIT   NUTS   WHOLE GRAINS

Energy Level   1   2   3   4   5   6   7   8   9   10

MOVEMENT

Time of Day   Comments

Walking ——————— steps/minutes

Weights   ——————— lbs, ——— reps

Stretches ——————— minutes

Laughter   ———————

Other   ————————————————————————   **Weight** ———————————

BLOOD GLUCOSE NUMBERS

Time	Breakfast Before	Breakfast After	Lunch Before	Lunch After	Dinner Before	Dinner After	Bedtime

MEDICATIONS

Time	Type

Carbohydrates Count

Carbohydrate raises your blood glucose after you eat it. Carbohydrate is found in grains, breads, desserts, fruits, vegetables, and beans. People with diabetes focus on the carb in their meals so they can bring their blood glucose back down. People on certain diets also focus on carb. You can use carb counting books to get the amount of carb in foods. A piece of fruit has about 15 grams of carbohydrate, or 1 carbohydrate choice. A meal plan based on carbs may give you 3 carb choices at breakfast, 4 at lunch, and 5 at dinner. That is 45 grams of carb at breakfast ($3 \times 15 = 45$), 60 grams at lunch, and 75 at dinner. You can choose among many foods to fit into the meal. A glass of milk is 12 grams of carb, a piece of toast is 15 grams of carb. You see how you can put your meal together by choosing from the many carb-containing foods? One key is to know what your choices are and then to make decisions that support a healthy lifestyle.

—**Marion Franz, RD, MS**
Director of Nutrition, International Diabetes Center, Minneapolis
www.idcdiabetes.org

Date _____ Deep Breathing _____ Sleep _____
HOURS

Water ⊔ ⊔ ⊔ ⊔ ⊔ ⊔ ⊔ ⊔   Blood Pressure _____

F O O D

BREAKFAST   Time _____ Total Carb_____

          Serving Size   Food and Drinks

Grain
Vegetable
Protein
Fruit
Milk
Fat

SNACK   Time _____ Total Carb_____

LUNCH   Time _____ Total Carb_____

          Serving Size   Food and Drinks

Grain
Vegetable
Protein
Fruit
Milk
Fat

SNACK   Time _____ Total Carb_____

DINNER   Time _____ Total Carb_____

          Serving Size   Food and Drinks

Grain
Vegetable
Protein
Fruit
Milk
Fat

TOTALS

VEGETABLES   FRUIT   NUTS   WHOLE GRAINS

FUN	EMOTIONS	MOOD	ILLNESS	STRESS

Energy Level 1 2 3 4 5 6 7 8 9 10

MOVEMENT

Time of Day   Comments

Walking _____ steps/minutes

Weights _____ lbs, _____ reps

Stretches _____ minutes

Laughter _____

Other _____   **Weight** _____

	BLOOD GLUCOSE NUMBERS								MEDICATIONS	
	Breakfast		Lunch		Dinner				Time	Type
Time	Before	After	Before	After	Before	After	Bedtime			

A Healthy Diet Chosen from Many Foods

- Can cut the risk of diseases, especially heart disease, diabetes, and cancer.
- Helps you feel better and have more energy.

Who can help you design a meal plan? A registered dietitian (RD) is trained in nutrition and can teach you about healthy eating. Contact your local hospital and ask for a dietitian or contact The American Dietetic Association at 1-800-366-1655 or www.eatright.org

- Look at the Nutrition Facts food label, and find the serving size.
- Limit yourself to a single serving of each food you choose.
- Work with an RD to establish your calorie goal.
- Look at your food records with the RD to understand your needs and usual food choices, and discover where and how to make better choices.
- Measure unfamiliar foods so you can see what an actual portion is.

—Ann Gallagher, RD
Former President, American Dietetic Association

Date _____ Deep Breathing _____ Sleep _____
HOURS

Water ▯ ▯ ▯ ▯ ▯ ▯ ▯ ▯   Blood Pressure _____

F O O D

BREAKFAST   Time _____ Total Carb_____

      Serving Size   Food and Drinks

Grain
Vegetable
Protein
Fruit
Milk
Fat

SNACK   Time _____ Total Carb_____

LUNCH   Time _____ Total Carb_____

      Serving Size   Food and Drinks

Grain
Vegetable
Protein
Fruit
Milk
Fat

SNACK   Time _____ Total Carb_____

DINNER   Time _____ Total Carb_____

      Serving Size   Food and Drinks

Grain
Vegetable
Protein
Fruit
Milk
Fat

T O T A L S

VEGETABLES   FRUIT   NUTS   WHOLE GRAINS

FUN	EMOTIONS	MOOD	ILLNESS	STRESS

Energy Level   1   2   3   4   5   6   7   8   9   10

MOVEMENT

Time of Day   Comments

Walking _____ steps/minutes

Weights _____ lbs, _____ reps

Stretches _____ minutes

Laughter _____

Other _____   **Weight** _____

BLOOD GLUCOSE NUMBERS

Time	Breakfast		Lunch		Dinner		Bedtime
	Before	After	Before	After	Before	After	

MEDICATIONS

Time	Type

The Ways and Whys We Eat

The meaning of food: Food is survival, like putting gas in the car, the car won't run without it; food is a friend and a comfort; food can be an escape, almost a lover of sorts, as people look forward to time alone with food; food is our culture and the way we were raised. Because we eat often, eating habits may be difficult to break.

You can learn to reshape habits that lead to obesity or binge eating. Make strategies for dining out: order appetizers instead of entrées, halve an entrée with a friend, or take half home for lunch tomorrow. Set small goals you can build on to create success.

The meaning of moderation: "not too much or too little of a variety of foods."

What about foods that make it difficult to practice moderation? Look at the portion size on the label, take one serving and put the rest back. Some people can eat just a little of the foods they crave; others must just stay away from these foods.

—Paul Garfinkel, MD
Chief of Psychiatry, University of Toronto

Date _____ Deep Breathing _____ Sleep _____
HOURS

Water ☐ ☐ ☐ ☐ ☐ ☐ ☐ ☐ Blood Pressure _____

F O O D

BREAKFAST Time _____ Total Carb_____

Serving Size Food and Drinks

Grain
Vegetable
Protein
Fruit
Milk
Fat

SNACK Time _____ Total Carb_____

LUNCH Time _____ Total Carb_____

Serving Size Food and Drinks

Grain
Vegetable
Protein
Fruit
Milk
Fat

SNACK Time _____ Total Carb_____

DINNER Time _____ Total Carb_____

Serving Size Food and Drinks

Grain
Vegetable
Protein
Fruit
Milk
Fat

T O T A L S

VEGETABLES   FRUIT   NUTS   WHOLE GRAINS

FUN	EMOTIONS	MOOD	ILLNESS	STRESS

Energy Level 1 2 3 4 5 6 7 8 9 10

MOVEMENT

Time of Day   Comments

Walking _____ steps/minutes

Weights _____ lbs, _____ reps

Stretches _____ minutes

Laughter _____

Other _____   **Weight** _____

BLOOD GLUCOSE NUMBERS							
	Breakfast		Lunch		Dinner		
Time	Before	After	Before	After	Before	After	Bedtime

MEDICATIONS	
Time	Type

Weight Loss Counts

National Weight Registry (Call 1-800-606-NWCR)

Why take action if you are overweight?

If people stop overeating, we can prevent over 300,000 deaths a year in North America.

Key weight loss strategies:

- Select low-fat foods (24% of calories from fat a day).
- Limit total calories in addition to a low-fat diet.
- Exercise. It burns calories, so you don't have to be so concerned about every little thing you eat. Exercise 60–90 minutes a day.
- Keep track of your weight and food so you see problems early, and develop a strategy to correct a problem before it turns into a habit.
- Plan ahead so you can make healthy food choices.
- Exercise is as important as eating, and it can be done throughout the day, too.

—James Hill, PhD
Director, Colorado Clinical Research Unit
Holly Thompson-Wyatt, MD, Univerity of Colorado

Date _____ Deep Breathing _____ Sleep _____

HOURS

Water ⊔ ⊔ ⊔ ⊔ ⊔ ⊔ ⊔ ⊔   Blood Pressure _____

F O O D

BREAKFAST   Time _____ Total Carb_____

       Serving Size   Food and Drinks

Grain
Vegetable
Protein
Fruit
Milk
Fat

SNACK   Time _____ Total Carb_____

LUNCH   Time _____ Total Carb_____

       Serving Size   Food and Drinks

Grain
Vegetable
Protein
Fruit
Milk
Fat

SNACK   Time _____ Total Carb_____

DINNER   Time _____ Total Carb_____

       Serving Size   Food and Drinks

Grain
Vegetable
Protein
Fruit
Milk
Fat

T O T A L S

VEGETABLES   FRUIT   NUTS   WHOLE GRAINS

FUN	EMOTIONS	MOOD	ILLNESS	STRESS

Energy Level 1 2 3 4 5 6 7 8 9 10

MOVEMENT

Time of Day   Comments

Walking _____ steps/minutes

Weights _____ lbs, _____ reps

Stretches _____ minutes

Laughter _____

Other _____   **Weight** _____

BLOOD GLUCOSE NUMBERS							
	Breakfast		Lunch		Dinner		
Time	Before	After	Before	After	Before	After	Bedtime

MEDICATIONS	
Time	Type

Key Strategies to Manage Stress

- The goal is not to eliminate stress but to aim for a middle ground.
- Keep a diary of stress (creates a self-awareness).
- Problem-solve—work through areas that appear to be most stressful.
- Exercise is a wonderful stress reducer and great for your health. A walk helps you sort things through; yoga or stretching helps relax tense muscles.
- A study of executives showed that taking brief breaks resulted in reduced absence at work and reduced stress.
- Deep breathing relaxes the body and gives you a break anywhere, anytime.
- Medicine may be necessary when strategies are not enough. You have not failed, you're just being able to control your health and giving the strategies time to work.

Find ways to manage stress that are transparent (become an everyday part of your life), which will lead to your success.

—Jeff Janata, PhD
Psychologist, University Hospitals of Cleveland

Date _____ Deep Breathing _____ Sleep _____

HOURS

Water ☐ ☐ ☐ ☐ ☐ ☐ ☐ ☐   Blood Pressure _____

F O O D

BREAKFAST
Time _____ Total Carb_____

Serving Size   Food and Drinks

Grain
Vegetable
Protein
Fruit
Milk
Fat

SNACK
Time _____ Total Carb_____

LUNCH
Time _____ Total Carb_____

Serving Size   Food and Drinks

Grain
Vegetable
Protein
Fruit
Milk
Fat

SNACK
Time _____ Total Carb_____

DINNER
Time _____ Total Carb_____

Serving Size   Food and Drinks

Grain
Vegetable
Protein
Fruit
Milk
Fat

T O T A L S

VEGETABLES   FRUIT   NUTS   WHOLE GRAINS

Energy Level 1 2 3 4 5 6 7 8 9 10

MOVEMENT

Time of Day   Comments

Walking _____ steps/minutes

Weights _____ lbs, _____ reps

Stretches _____ minutes

Laughter _____

Other _____

Weight _____

BLOOD GLUCOSE NUMBERS

Time	Breakfast		Lunch		Dinner		Bedtime
	Before	After	Before	After	Before	After	

MEDICATIONS

Time	Type

Stress

Stress affects our bodies and behavior through the "fight or flight" hormones, which are powerful. Research on medical students (highly stressed folks) shows that the stress of exams affects the immune system. People are much more susceptible to illness, colds, and flu while under stress. Stress can influence blood sugar levels, too. People under stress are not even-tempered and can't think clearly. Stress impairs our ability to function and makes us irritable.

What Can You Do about Stress?

- Exercise, eat well, and learn what makes you well.
- Stress management counseling provides tools to make the best choices for health.
- Find exercise that you enjoy and do often; it will positively affect your stress level.

Remember, some stress is a good thing and can challenge us to make positive healthy choices!

—Jeff Janata, PhD
Psychologist, University Hospitals of Cleveland

Date _____ Deep Breathing _____ Sleep _____
HOURS

Water ⊔ ⊔ ⊔ ⊔ ⊔ ⊔ ⊔ ⊔   Blood Pressure _____

F O O D

BREAKFAST   Time _____ Total Carb_____

	Serving Size	Food and Drinks
Grain		
Vegetable		
Protein		
Fruit		
Milk		
Fat		

SNACK   Time _____ Total Carb_____

LUNCH   Time _____ Total Carb_____

	Serving Size	Food and Drinks
Grain		
Vegetable		
Protein		
Fruit		
Milk		
Fat		

SNACK   Time _____ Total Carb_____

DINNER   Time _____ Total Carb_____

	Serving Size	Food and Drinks
Grain		
Vegetable		
Protein		
Fruit		
Milk		
Fat		

T O T A L S

VEGETABLES   FRUIT   NUTS   WHOLE GRAINS

| FUN | EMOTIONS | MOOD | ILLNESS | STRESS |

Energy Level 1 2 3 4 5 6 7 8 9 10

MOVEMENT

Time of Day   Comments

Walking _____ steps/minutes

Weights _____ lbs, _____ reps

Stretches _____ minutes

Laughter _____

Other _____

Weight _____

BLOOD GLUCOSE NUMBERS

Time	Breakfast Before	Breakfast After	Lunch Before	Lunch After	Dinner Before	Dinner After	Bedtime

MEDICATIONS

Time	Type

Fats

Fats: You need some fat in your meals, but all fats are high in calories, so find out which ones help you the most.

Saturated fat is solid at room temperature, as in butter or margarine. Animal fats and tropical oils like coconut and palm oil are saturated fats. This kind of fat raises your cholesterol level. That's why you don't want to eat too much of it.

Unsaturated fats are fluid at room temperature. You find them in plants and fish—flax, sunflower, and sesame seeds; nuts; olives; fish; and olive, canola, and peanut oils. Unsaturated fat lowers LDL (bad) cholesterol and protects the HDL (good) cholesterol. This is why these fats are good for your body.

Don't eliminate butter from your diet, because it tastes great, and oftentimes, you must cook with butter to get the right flavor. The trans fats in margarine sticks are saturated fats, so butter is just as good. But most of the time, choose olive or canola oil.

—Peter Jones, PhD
Director, Human Nutrition Program, McGill University

Date _____ Deep Breathing _____ Sleep _____
HOURS

Water ⬜ ⬜ ⬜ ⬜ ⬜ ⬜ ⬜ ⬜   Blood Pressure _____

F O O D

BREAKFAST
Time _____ Total Carb_____

Serving Size Food and Drinks

Grain
Vegetable
Protein
Fruit
Milk
Fat

SNACK
Time _____ Total Carb_____

LUNCH
Time _____ Total Carb_____

Serving Size Food and Drinks

Grain
Vegetable
Protein
Fruit
Milk
Fat

SNACK
Time _____ Total Carb_____

DINNER
Time _____ Total Carb_____

Serving Size Food and Drinks

Grain
Vegetable
Protein
Fruit
Milk
Fat

T O T A L S

VEGETABLES   FRUIT   NUTS   WHOLE GRAINS

| FUN | EMOTIONS | MOOD | ILLNESS | STRESS |

Energy Level 1 2 3 4 5 6 7 8 9 10

MOVEMENT

Time of Day   Comments

Walking _____ steps/minutes

Weights _____ lbs, _____ reps

Stretches _____ minutes

Laughter _____

Other _____ **Weight** _____

BLOOD GLUCOSE NUMBERS							
	Breakfast		Lunch		Dinner		
Time	Before	After	Before	After	Before	After	Bedtime

MEDICATIONS	
Time	Type

Roasting Red Peppers

GRAHAM

Cut off both ends of the pepper and run a blade around the inside to remove the seeds; cut the remaining pepper into four sections and place them flat on a broiler pan, with the skin up. Broil until the peppers are blackened. Place the peppers into a bag, which retains the heat and helps the skin to separate from the flesh.

Date _____ Deep Breathing _____ Sleep _____
HOURS

Water ▯ ▯ ▯ ▯ ▯ ▯ ▯ ▯   Blood Pressure _____

F O O D

BREAKFAST
Time _____ Total Carb_____

Serving Size	Food and Drinks
Grain	
Vegetable	
Protein	
Fruit	
Milk	
Fat	

SNACK
Time _____ Total Carb_____

LUNCH
Time _____ Total Carb_____

Serving Size	Food and Drinks
Grain	
Vegetable	
Protein	
Fruit	
Milk	
Fat	

SNACK
Time _____ Total Carb_____

DINNER
Time _____ Total Carb_____

Serving Size	Food and Drinks
Grain	
Vegetable	
Protein	
Fruit	
Milk	
Fat	

T O T A L S

VEGETABLES   FRUIT   NUTS   WHOLE GRAINS

FUN	EMOTIONS	MOOD	ILLNESS	STRESS

Energy Level 1 2 3 4 5 6 7 8 9 10

MOVEMENT

Time of Day   Comments

Walking _____ steps/minutes

Weights _____ lbs, _____ reps

Stretches _____ minutes

Laughter _____

Other _____   **Weight** _____

BLOOD GLUCOSE NUMBERS

Time	Breakfast		Lunch		Dinner		Bedtime
	Before	After	Before	After	Before	After	

MEDICATIONS

Time	Type

African American Health Concerns

Health concerns for the African American population:

- Obesity
- Diabetes
- High blood pressure

These health problems are all caused by diet choices: saturated fat; too many calories; lack of fiber from fruits, vegetables, and whole grains; and too large serving sizes. These health problems can be improved by making better dietary choices.

Exercise is another key to better health:

- Helps to lower blood pressure.
- Helps control diabetes.
- Is important for weight loss and weight maintenance.
- Can be done in short intervals during the day and still get the benefit.

—Jeannette Jordan, MS, RD, CDE
Education Coordinator, Medical University of South Carolina
Author, *Good Health Cookbook*

Date _____ Deep Breathing _____ Sleep _____
HOURS

Water ⊔ ⊔ ⊔ ⊔ ⊔ ⊔ ⊔ ⊔   Blood Pressure _____

F O O D

BREAKFAST   Time _____ Total Carb_____

          Serving Size   Food and Drinks
Grain
Vegetable
Protein
Fruit
Milk
Fat

SNACK   Time _____ Total Carb_____

LUNCH   Time _____ Total Carb_____

          Serving Size   Food and Drinks
Grain
Vegetable
Protein
Fruit
Milk
Fat

SNACK   Time _____ Total Carb_____

DINNER   Time _____ Total Carb_____

          Serving Size   Food and Drinks
Grain
Vegetable
Protein
Fruit
Milk
Fat

T O T A L S

VEGETABLES   FRUIT   NUTS   WHOLE GRAINS

FUN	EMOTIONS	MOOD	ILLNESS	STRESS

Energy Level 1 2 3 4 5 6 7 8 9 10

MOVEMENT

Time of Day   Comments

Walking _____ steps/minutes

Weights _____ lbs, _____ reps

Stretches _____ minutes

Laughter _____

Other _____   **Weight** _____

BLOOD GLUCOSE NUMBERS								MEDICATIONS	
	Breakfast		Lunch		Dinner			Time	Type
Time	Before	After	Before	After	Before	After	Bedtime		

To Lose Weight Use Your Head

Spot reduction does not work! Move your whole body as often as possible. Find enjoyable ways to move the large muscles in your arms and legs, and remember that if weight loss is your goal, whole body exercises are best for burning calories, too.

Research shows there is no selective use of calories by various parts of the body, instead calories are utilized by the body as a whole. Also, no additional weight is lost from certain areas of the body just because of more muscle tone. Even 5,000 sit-ups won't result in more weight loss in the stomach versus the arm.

—Victor L. Katch, PhD
University of Michigan
Author, *The Fidget Factor and Exercise Physiology*

Date _____ Deep Breathing _____ Sleep _____
HOURS

Water ⬜ ⬜ ⬜ ⬜ ⬜ ⬜ ⬜ ⬜ Blood Pressure _____

F O O D

BREAKFAST Time _____ Total Carb_____

Serving Size   Food and Drinks

Grain
Vegetable
Protein
Fruit
Milk
Fat

SNACK Time _____ Total Carb_____

LUNCH Time _____ Total Carb_____

Serving Size   Food and Drinks

Grain
Vegetable
Protein
Fruit
Milk
Fat

SNACK Time _____ Total Carb_____

DINNER Time _____ Total Carb_____

Serving Size   Food and Drinks

Grain
Vegetable
Protein
Fruit
Milk
Fat

T O T A L S

VEGETABLES   FRUIT   NUTS   WHOLE GRAINS

FUN	EMOTIONS	MOOD	ILLNESS	STRESS

Energy Level   1   2   3   4   5   6   7   8   9   10

MOVEMENT

Time of Day   Comments

Walking _____ steps/minutes

Weights _____ lbs, _____ reps

Stretches _____ minutes

Laughter _____

Other _____   **Weight** _____

BLOOD GLUCOSE NUMBERS

Time	Breakfast		Lunch		Dinner		Bedtime
	Before	After	Before	After	Before	After	

MEDICATIONS

Time	Type

Exercise Burns Calories

The most effective way to lose weight is a combination of decreasing calories you eat and increasing the number of calories you burn, or, more exercise and less food. Exercise burns calories as you do it, but it also speeds up metabolism so that you burn more calories even at rest than you would have had you not exercised at all.

As we lose weight, fat comes off the whole body beginning with the largest fat-containing area. Most body fat is located in the abdominal area. However, there are five major fat deposits on the body and fat accrues in these areas as we age.

Goal: Exercise to be in the best of health.

Approach: Exercise daily and fidget often. Expend 300 calories a day through exercise. Walk about 3 miles a day (about 30–45 minutes). People who "fidget" (extra movements while sitting or standing) can lose 8–12 pounds a year.

—**Victor L. Katch, PhD**
University of Michigan
Author, *The Fidget Factor and Exercise Physiology*

Date _____ Deep Breathing _____ Sleep _____
HOURS

Water ☐ ☐ ☐ ☐ ☐ ☐ ☐ ☐   Blood Pressure _____

F O O D

BREAKFAST   Time _____ Total Carb_____

      Serving Size   Food and Drinks

Grain
Vegetable
Protein
Fruit
Milk
Fat

SNACK   Time _____ Total Carb_____

LUNCH   Time _____ Total Carb_____

      Serving Size   Food and Drinks

Grain
Vegetable
Protein
Fruit
Milk
Fat

SNACK   Time _____ Total Carb_____

DINNER   Time _____ Total Carb_____

      Serving Size   Food and Drinks

Grain
Vegetable
Protein
Fruit
Milk
Fat

T O T A L S

VEGETABLES   FRUIT   NUTS   WHOLE GRAINS

FUN	EMOTIONS	MOOD	ILLNESS	STRESS

Energy Level 1 2 3 4 5 6 7 8 9 10

MOVEMENT

Time of Day   Comments

Walking _____ steps/minutes

Weights _____ lbs, _____ reps

Stretches _____ minutes

Laughter _____

Other _____   Weight _____

BLOOD GLUCOSE NUMBERS

Time	Breakfast		Lunch		Dinner		Bedtime
	Before	After	Before	After	Before	After	

MEDICATIONS

Time	Type

Healthy Insight for the Day

GRAHAM

Try this yummy yogurt cheese spread recipe:

Turn a 32-oz container of plain nonfat yogurt (no cornstarch or thickeners) into a strainer/colander that is set into a large bowl containing absorbent kitchen toweling. Place in the refrigerator for at least 8 hours or overnight.

The whey drains away, and you are left with a thick yogurt cheese.

Mix in equal proportions with soft (tub) light margarine (with no trans fatty acids) to create a spread for English muffins or toast. You can use 2/3 yogurt and 1/3 margarine for less fat and calories.

Mix with maple syrup to serve alongside a slice of pie or top a baked potato with ground pepper, chives, and yogurt cheese.

Date _____ Deep Breathing _____ Sleep _____
                                                                    HOURS
Water ⬓ ⬓ ⬓ ⬓ ⬓ ⬓ ⬓ ⬓   Blood Pressure _____

F O O D

BREAKFAST   Time _____ Total Carb _____

      Serving Size   Food and Drinks

Grain
Vegetable
Protein
Fruit
Milk
Fat

SNACK   Time _____ Total Carb _____

LUNCH   Time _____ Total Carb _____

      Serving Size   Food and Drinks

Grain
Vegetable
Protein
Fruit
Milk
Fat

SNACK   Time _____ Total Carb _____

DINNER   Time _____ Total Carb _____

      Serving Size   Food and Drinks

Grain
Vegetable
Protein
Fruit
Milk
Fat

T O T A L S

VEGETABLES   FRUIT   NUTS   WHOLE GRAINS

Energy Level   1   2   3   4   5   6   7   8   9   10

MOVEMENT

Time of Day   Comments

Walking _____ steps/minutes

Weights _____ lbs, _____ reps

Stretches _____ minutes

Laughter _____

Other _____   Weight _____

BLOOD GLUCOSE NUMBERS

Time	Breakfast		Lunch		Dinner		Bedtime
	Before	After	Before	After	Before	After	

MEDICATIONS

Time	Type

Healthy Insight for the Day

GRAHAM

Here are six easy ways to eliminate processed carbohydrates:

Cut your portions of bread, jam, and sugar at breakfast in half.

Minimize bread at lunch by having an open-faced sandwich.

Replace snacks like pretzels or chips with a fresh fruit or vegetable.

Cut down on snacks like fig newtons, fat-free cookies, and sweets.

Halve portions of pasta or rice at mealtimes.

Eliminate a high-calorie snack and choose water and a walk instead.

Dinner Parties are a way you can gather around the table and share in the preparation as well as the enjoyment of the meal. Have each person make a different course, which will ease the amount of work for everyone.

Date _____ Deep Breathing _____ Sleep _____
HOURS

Water ☐ ☐ ☐ ☐ ☐ ☐ ☐ ☐   Blood Pressure _____

F O O D

BREAKFAST   Time _____ Total Carb_____

      Serving Size   Food and Drinks

Grain
Vegetable
Protein
Fruit
Milk
Fat

SNACK   Time _____ Total Carb_____

LUNCH   Time _____ Total Carb_____

      Serving Size   Food and Drinks

Grain
Vegetable
Protein
Fruit
Milk
Fat

SNACK   Time _____ Total Carb_____

DINNER   Time _____ Total Carb_____

      Serving Size   Food and Drinks

Grain
Vegetable
Protein
Fruit
Milk
Fat

T O T A L S

VEGETABLES   FRUIT   NUTS   WHOLE GRAINS

FUN	EMOTIONS	MOOD	ILLNESS	STRESS

Energy Level   1   2   3   4   5   6   7   8   9   10

MOVEMENT

Time of Day   Comments

Walking _____ steps/minutes

Weights _____ lbs, _____ reps

Stretches _____ minutes

Laughter _____

Other _____   **Weight** _____

BLOOD GLUCOSE NUMBERS

| Time | Breakfast | | Lunch | | Dinner | | Bedtime |
	Before	After	Before	After	Before	After	

MEDICATIONS

Time	Type

Healthy Insight for the Day

GRAHAM

Top ten picks for fiber (we need 20–30 grams a day):

1 Orange	7 grams
1/2 Grapefruit	6 grams
Broccoli	5 grams per serving
Spinach	5 grams per serving
Apples	5 grams per serving
Bananas	4 grams per serving
Sweet potatoes	4 grams per serving
Strawberries	4 grams per serving
Kiwifruit	4 grams per serving
Leaf lettuce	4 grams per serving

What are your favorite fiber-filled foods?

Date _____ Deep Breathing _____ Sleep _____
HOURS

Water ⬜ ⬜ ⬜ ⬜ ⬜ ⬜ ⬜ ⬜   Blood Pressure _____

F O O D

BREAKFAST   Time _____ Total Carb _____

       Serving Size   Food and Drinks

Grain
Vegetable
Protein
Fruit
Milk
Fat

SNACK   Time _____ Total Carb _____

LUNCH   Time _____ Total Carb _____

       Serving Size   Food and Drinks

Grain
Vegetable
Protein
Fruit
Milk
Fat

SNACK   Time _____ Total Carb _____

DINNER   Time _____ Total Carb _____

       Serving Size   Food and Drinks

Grain
Vegetable
Protein
Fruit
Milk
Fat

TOTALS

VEGETABLES   FRUIT   NUTS   WHOLE GRAINS

Energy Level   1   2   3   4   5   6   7   8   9   10

MOVEMENT

Time of Day   Comments

Walking _____ steps/minutes

Weights _____ lbs, _____ reps

Stretches _____ minutes

Laughter _____

Other _____   Weight _____

BLOOD GLUCOSE NUMBERS

| Time | Breakfast | | Lunch | | Dinner | | Bedtime |
	Before	After	Before	After	Before	After	

MEDICATIONS

Time	Type

Healthy Insight for the Day

GRAHAM

You decide which road you would like to take.

Road to Reversal: If you are sick or you are taking care of someone who is sick and would like to be well, try eating <10% of calories from fat and mostly vegetarian meals.

Road to Prevention: If you are well and don't want to get sick, try 20% of calories from fat, more vegetables and less meat, say 3 1/2 oz of meat a day.

Same Old Road: If you are not interested in making any choices/changes about your health (you probably aren't reading this book), you get to choose to proceed through the intersection without making any changes at all.

Goal: Consider one or two days a week that you will prepare vegetarian meals without chicken, pork, or beef regardless of your health needs.

Consult your doctor and registered dietitian for recommendations that are individualized to meet your needs.

Date _____ Deep Breathing _____ Sleep _____
HOURS

Water ⎕ ⎕ ⎕ ⎕ ⎕ ⎕ ⎕ ⎕   Blood Pressure _____

F O O D

BREAKFAST   Time _____ Total Carb_____

      Serving Size   Food and Drinks

Grain
Vegetable
Protein
Fruit
Milk
Fat

SNACK   Time _____ Total Carb_____

LUNCH   Time _____ Total Carb_____

      Serving Size   Food and Drinks

Grain
Vegetable
Protein
Fruit
Milk
Fat

SNACK   Time _____ Total Carb_____

DINNER   Time _____ Total Carb_____

      Serving Size   Food and Drinks

Grain
Vegetable
Protein
Fruit
Milk
Fat

T O T A L S

VEGETABLES   FRUIT   NUTS   WHOLE GRAINS

Energy Level   1   2   3   4   5   6   7   8   9   10

MOVEMENT

Time of Day   Comments

Walking _____ steps/minutes

Weights _____ lbs, _____ reps

Stretches _____ minutes

Laughter _____

Other _____   Weight _____

BLOOD GLUCOSE NUMBERS							
	Breakfast		Lunch		Dinner		
Time	Before	After	Before	After	Before	After	Bedtime

MEDICATIONS	
Time	Type

Healthy Insight for the Day

GRAHAM

To calculate a target body weight, try this general guideline:

For women, allow 100 pounds for the first five feet. For every inch over five feet, add five pounds. If a woman is 5 feet, 5 inches tall, her target weight would be 125 pounds.

For men, allow 106 pounds for the first five feet. For every inch over five feet, add six pounds. If a male is six feet tall, he would have a target weight of 178 pounds.

(Add 10% for a large frame and subtract 10% for a small frame.)

Please consult with a qualified health professional to help you identify an ideal target weight for you!

A healthy weight may not be a "pretty" or fashionable weight. It is the weight where all your health measures—blood pressure, blood sugar, and cholesterol—are normal.

Date _____ Deep Breathing _____ Sleep _____
                                                              HOURS
Water ⬚ ⬚ ⬚ ⬚ ⬚ ⬚ ⬚ ⬚   Blood Pressure _____

F O O D

BREAKFAST   Time _____ Total Carb_____

	Serving Size	Food and Drinks
Grain		
Vegetable		
Protein		
Fruit		
Milk		
Fat		

SNACK   Time _____ Total Carb_____

LUNCH   Time _____ Total Carb_____

	Serving Size	Food and Drinks
Grain		
Vegetable		
Protein		
Fruit		
Milk		
Fat		

SNACK   Time _____ Total Carb_____

DINNER   Time _____ Total Carb_____

	Serving Size	Food and Drinks
Grain		
Vegetable		
Protein		
Fruit		
Milk		
Fat		

TOTALS

VEGETABLES   FRUIT   NUTS   WHOLE GRAINS

| FUN | EMOTIONS | MOOD | ILLNESS | STRESS |

Energy Level 1 2 3 4 5 6 7 8 9 10

MOVEMENT

Time of Day   Comments

Walking _____ steps/minutes

Weights _____ lbs, _____ reps

Stretches _____ minutes

Laughter _____

Other _____   **Weight** _____

BLOOD GLUCOSE NUMBERS								MEDICATIONS	
	Breakfast		Lunch		Dinner			Time	Type
Time	Before	After	Before	After	Before	After	Bedtime		

Healthy Insight for the Day

GRAHAM

To estimate the number of calories you need, try this:

Multiply your weight by the activity factor based on your age (see chart below) to find your caloric level to maintain your weight.

_____ (lbs) × _____ (AF) = _____ calories

Activity Factor
Age 20–30: 13–15

Age 30–40: 12

Age 40–50: 11

Age 50 plus: 10 (As we age, our metabolism slows!)

For weight loss, subtract 250 calories daily, and for weight gain add 250 calories daily. In a week's time, if you subtract 250 calories a day, you can lose up to one pound. Or by adding the calories, you will gain a pound.

Date _____ Deep Breathing _____ Sleep _____
HOURS

Water ⊔ ⊔ ⊔ ⊔ ⊔ ⊔ ⊔ ⊔ Blood Pressure _____

F O O D

BREAKFAST　　　　　Time _____ Total Carb_____

　　　　Serving Size　　Food and Drinks

Grain
Vegetable
Protein
Fruit
Milk
Fat

SNACK　　　　　　　Time _____ Total Carb_____

LUNCH　　　　　　　Time _____ Total Carb_____

　　　　Serving Size　　Food and Drinks

Grain
Vegetable
Protein
Fruit
Milk
Fat

SNACK　　　　　　　Time _____ Total Carb_____

DINNER　　　　　　Time _____ Total Carb_____

　　　　Serving Size　　Food and Drinks

Grain
Vegetable
Protein
Fruit
Milk
Fat

TOTALS

VEGETABLES　　　　　FRUIT　　　　NUTS　　　WHOLE GRAINS

FUN	EMOTIONS	MOOD	ILLNESS	STRESS

Energy Level 1 2 3 4 5 6 7 8 9 10

MOVEMENT

Time of Day   Comments

Walking _____ steps/minutes

Weights _____ lbs, _____ reps

Stretches _____ minutes

Laughter _____

Other _____   **Weight** _____

BLOOD GLUCOSE NUMBERS

Time	Breakfast		Lunch		Dinner		Bedtime
	Before	After	Before	After	Before	After	

MEDICATIONS

Time	Type

Healthy Insight for the Day

GRAHAM

If you've been asked to limit fat for better health or you simply want to cut back, try this:

Calories	20% Fat	25% Fat	30% Fat
1,200	25 grams	30 grams	40 grams
1,500	30 grams	40 grams	50 grams
2,000	40 grams	50 grams	65 grams
2,500	50 grams	65 grams	80 grams

When you know your weight, total cholesterol, LDL cholesterol, HDL cholesterol, triglycerides, your blood sugar, and blood pressure, you and your physician can determine your health risk. When you understand your risk of developing a health problem, you will more fully understand what you need to do to be well.

Date _____ Deep Breathing _____ Sleep _____
HOURS

Water ⬜ ⬜ ⬜ ⬜ ⬜ ⬜ ⬜ ⬜   Blood Pressure _____

F O O D

BREAKFAST   Time _____ Total Carb_____

　　　　　Serving Size   Food and Drinks

Grain
Vegetable
Protein
Fruit
Milk
Fat

SNACK   Time _____ Total Carb_____

LUNCH   Time _____ Total Carb_____

　　　　　Serving Size   Food and Drinks

Grain
Vegetable
Protein
Fruit
Milk
Fat

SNACK   Time _____ Total Carb_____

DINNER   Time _____ Total Carb_____

　　　　　Serving Size   Food and Drinks

Grain
Vegetable
Protein
Fruit
Milk
Fat

TOTALS

VEGETABLES　　　　　FRUIT　　　NUTS　　　WHOLE GRAINS

FUN	EMOTIONS	MOOD	ILLNESS	STRESS

Energy Level   1   2   3   4   5   6   7   8   9   10

MOVEMENT

Time of Day   Comments

Walking _____ steps/minutes

Weights _____ lbs, _____ reps

Stretches _____ minutes

Laughter _____

Other _____ **Weight** _____

BLOOD GLUCOSE NUMBERS							
	Breakfast		Lunch		Dinner		
Time	Before	After	Before	After	Before	After	Bedtime

MEDICATIONS	
Time	Type

Healthy Insight for the Day

What techniques are used in any kitchen to make food delicious and nutritious?

- Use fresh foods. Salads are fresh with fresh fruits and veggies and fat-free dressings.
- Serve the freshest seasonal fruit.
- Select lean meats and prepare them healthfully, with herbs and spices.
- Meats are served with salsas, slaws, and purees.
- Meat is served in 3–4-oz portion and paired with vegetables on half the plate and starches on one-quarter of the plate.
- Healthy oils are used—olive and canola oils.
- Enhance vegetables with herbs, stocks, and aromatics, such as onions and garlic.
- Low-fat dairy products are used.
- Menus feature plant-based entrees, vegetarian fare.
- Serve a variety of foods at every meal.

—Mary Kimbrough, RD, LD
Director, Nutrition Services, Zale Lipshy University Hospital

Date _____ Deep Breathing _____ Sleep _____
HOURS

Water ⬚ ⬚ ⬚ ⬚ ⬚ ⬚ ⬚ ⬚   Blood Pressure _____

F O O D

BREAKFAST Time _____ Total Carb_____

    Serving Size   Food and Drinks

Grain
Vegetable
Protein
Fruit
Milk
Fat

SNACK Time _____ Total Carb_____

LUNCH Time _____ Total Carb_____

    Serving Size   Food and Drinks

Grain
Vegetable
Protein
Fruit
Milk
Fat

SNACK Time _____ Total Carb_____

DINNER Time _____ Total Carb_____

    Serving Size   Food and Drinks

Grain
Vegetable
Protein
Fruit
Milk
Fat

TOTALS

VEGETABLES   FRUIT   NUTS   WHOLE GRAINS

FUN	EMOTIONS	MOOD	ILLNESS	STRESS

Energy Level   1   2   3   4   5   6   7   8   9   10

MOVEMENT

Time of Day   Comments

Walking _____ steps/minutes

Weights _____ lbs, _____ reps

Stretches _____ minutes

Laughter _____

Other _____ **Weight** _____

BLOOD GLUCOSE NUMBERS

Time	Breakfast Before	Breakfast After	Lunch Before	Lunch After	Dinner Before	Dinner After	Bedtime

MEDICATIONS

Time	Type

Organic Farming

Organic farming is environmentally friendly and people friendly, too, because no toxins are applied directly to the foods as they grow or in ordinary food production. If you eat vegetables, fruit, and whole grains to be healthier—having them without poisons is even healthier.

If you buy locally and seasonally, organic foods are cost-effective. Look at your diet and choose organic foods for the greatest portion of what you eat; for example, if you eat a lot of potatoes, purchase organic potatoes.

How can we best make the change to organics?

- Look at what you eat the most of and buy the best quality organic food.
- Become aware of the food you are eating and read the labels.
- Look for certified organics—have a sticker or ask to see the papers on the food.
- If you don't know, ask to make sure it is organic.

Organic food is delicious. Taste-test it with a food you're eating now.

—Lorri King
Co-Owner Alternatives Organic Market

Date _____ Deep Breathing _____ Sleep _____
HOURS

Water ⬜ ⬜ ⬜ ⬜ ⬜ ⬜ ⬜ ⬜   Blood Pressure _____

F O O D

BREAKFAST
Time _____ Total Carb_____

	Serving Size	Food and Drinks
Grain		
Vegetable		
Protein		
Fruit		
Milk		
Fat		

SNACK
Time _____ Total Carb_____

LUNCH
Time _____ Total Carb_____

	Serving Size	Food and Drinks
Grain		
Vegetable		
Protein		
Fruit		
Milk		
Fat		

SNACK
Time _____ Total Carb_____

DINNER
Time _____ Total Carb_____

	Serving Size	Food and Drinks
Grain		
Vegetable		
Protein		
Fruit		
Milk		
Fat		

TOTALS

VEGETABLES   FRUIT   NUTS   WHOLE GRAINS

FUN	EMOTIONS	MOOD	ILLNESS	STRESS

Energy Level   1   2   3   4   5   6   7   8   9   10

MOVEMENT

Time of Day   Comments

Walking _____ steps/minutes

Weights _____ lbs, _____ reps

Stretches _____ minutes

Laughter _____

Other _____   **Weight** _____

BLOOD GLUCOSE NUMBERS								MEDICATIONS	
	Breakfast		Lunch		Dinner			Time	Type
Time	Before	After	Before	After	Before	After	Bedtime		

Healthy Insight for the Day

It is not only what you weigh, but where the fat is located on the body that defines your health risk. A bigger belly results in high cholesterol, high blood pressure, and heart disease, and a greater risk of diabetes and other serious diseases.

Be encouraged by small amounts of weight loss!
Small amounts of weight loss (5–10%) have dramatic benefits for your health.
Example: If a 154-pound person loses 5–10 pounds, it can lower blood pressure as much as medication for some people. It can bring blood sugar levels down, too. It can relieve joint pain and encourage you to make more healthy changes in your life.

—Lawrence Leiter, MD
Endocrinologist, St. Michael's Hospital
Associate Professor, Nutritional Sciences, University of Toronto

Date _____ Deep Breathing _____ Sleep _____
HOURS

Water ⊔ ⊔ ⊔ ⊔ ⊔ ⊔ ⊔ ⊔   Blood Pressure _____

F O O D

BREAKFAST   Time _____   Total Carb_____

          Serving Size   Food and Drinks
Grain
Vegetable
Protein
Fruit
Milk
Fat

SNACK   Time _____   Total Carb_____

LUNCH   Time _____   Total Carb_____

          Serving Size   Food and Drinks
Grain
Vegetable
Protein
Fruit
Milk
Fat

SNACK   Time _____   Total Carb_____

DINNER   Time _____   Total Carb_____

          Serving Size   Food and Drinks
Grain
Vegetable
Protein
Fruit
Milk
Fat

T O T A L S

VEGETABLES   FRUIT   NUTS   WHOLE GRAINS

FUN	EMOTIONS	MOOD	ILLNESS	STRESS

Energy Level 1 2 3 4 5 6 7 8 9 10

MOVEMENT

Time of Day   Comments

Walking _____ steps/minutes

Weights _____ lbs, _____ reps

Stretches _____ minutes

Laughter _____

Other _____   **Weight** _____

BLOOD GLUCOSE NUMBERS

Time	Breakfast		Lunch		Dinner		Bedtime
	Before	After	Before	After	Before	After	

MEDICATIONS

Time	Type

Are You Ready to Diet?

Often we know that something is right, but we don't do it. The challenge is to find a time when you are "diet ready" so change can take place, and you can be successful. Otherwise, it is often a waste of time. Sometimes, it takes a health crisis to make a person diet ready.

Any good thing takes time.
Realize that it takes time to lose weight. Set small goals for yourself, so they are manageable. For example, a goal of losing 1 pound a week would result in 50 pounds over the course of a year and 100 pounds in 2 years. Small steps for big rewards.

Make time for exercise.
Physical inactivity is one of the biggest problems we face. Find places to add regular activity to your day, because a simple daily walk can make a big difference.

—Lawrence Leiter, MD
Endocrinologist, St. Michael's Hospital
Associate Professor, Nutritional Sciences,
University of Toronto

Date _____ Deep Breathing _____ Sleep _____

HOURS

Water 🥛 🥛 🥛 🥛 🥛 🥛 🥛 🥛 Blood Pressure _____

F O O D

BREAKFAST
Time _____ Total Carb_____

Serving Size	Food and Drinks
Grain	
Vegetable	
Protein	
Fruit	
Milk	
Fat	

SNACK
Time _____ Total Carb_____

LUNCH
Time _____ Total Carb_____

Serving Size	Food and Drinks
Grain	
Vegetable	
Protein	
Fruit	
Milk	
Fat	

SNACK
Time _____ Total Carb_____

DINNER
Time _____ Total Carb_____

Serving Size	Food and Drinks
Grain	
Vegetable	
Protein	
Fruit	
Milk	
Fat	

TOTALS

VEGETABLES   FRUIT   NUTS   WHOLE GRAINS

FUN	EMOTIONS	MOOD	ILLNESS	STRESS

Energy Level 1 2 3 4 5 6 7 8 9 10

MOVEMENT

Time of Day   Comments

Walking _____ steps/minutes

Weights _____ lbs, _____ reps

Stretches _____ minutes

Laughter _____

Other _____   **Weight** _____

BLOOD GLUCOSE NUMBERS

Time	Breakfast		Lunch		Dinner		Bedtime
	Before	After	Before	After	Before	After	

MEDICATIONS

Time	Type

Sleep

Sleep deprivation (even small losses of sleep over time):

- Affects your mind, your concentration, and your reaction time
- Increases blood sugar levels
- Affects your sympathetic nervous system
- Causes aging overnight
- Can lead to early onset of type 2 diabetes, obesity, and hypertension

How much sleep do you need?
Keep track of the hours you sleep each night and how alert you are during the day. Most people have a mid-day dip in energy. Add 15-minute increments of sleep to the time you've been sleeping for a week until you're alert all day long. Most people need to add at least one more hour of sleep to their current sleep habits to feel alert all day long.

"When we move people from 7 to 8 hours of sleep, they all say after 12 weeks of going to bed earlier, they never knew what it was like to be awake!"

—James B. Maas, PhD
Professor of Psychology, Cornell University
Author, *Power Sleep*

Date _____ Deep Breathing _____ Sleep _____
HOURS

Water ⎕ ⎕ ⎕ ⎕ ⎕ ⎕ ⎕ ⎕   Blood Pressure _____

F O O D

BREAKFAST   Time _____ Total Carb_____

     Serving Size   Food and Drinks

Grain
Vegetable
Protein
Fruit
Milk
Fat

SNACK   Time _____ Total Carb_____

LUNCH   Time _____ Total Carb_____

     Serving Size   Food and Drinks

Grain
Vegetable
Protein
Fruit
Milk
Fat

SNACK   Time _____ Total Carb_____

DINNER   Time _____ Total Carb_____

     Serving Size   Food and Drinks

Grain
Vegetable
Protein
Fruit
Milk
Fat

T O T A L S

VEGETABLES   FRUIT   NUTS   WHOLE GRAINS

FUN	EMOTIONS	MOOD	ILLNESS	STRESS

Energy Level   1   2   3   4   5   6   7   8   9   10

MOVEMENT

Time of Day   Comments

Walking _____ steps/minutes

Weights _____ lbs, _____ reps

Stretches _____ minutes

Laughter _____

Other _____   **Weight** _____

BLOOD GLUCOSE NUMBERS

Time	Breakfast		Lunch		Dinner		Bedtime
	Before	After	Before	After	Before	After	

MEDICATIONS

Time	Type

Sleep Well

Wake up to these facts:

- Alertness increases by 25% when you add an hour of sleep to the 8 you already get.
- Don't sleep in on the weekends; this messes up your schedule. You have to be regular to get the best sleep; go to bed at the same time every day of the week.
- If you need an alarm to wake up, you are sleep deprived. If you fall asleep instantly, you are sleep starved. A well-rested person takes 15–20 minutes to fall asleep.
- Television and clocks with red LED display may disturb your sleep, so turn them off.
- The bedroom should be quiet, dark, and cool, about 65°F.
- Find a good pillow. Fold the pillow in half: if it springs forward by itself, it is fine; if not, get a new one.
- Make sure you have a great mattress—pocketed-coil springs are all separate.
- Write down or tape record your worries to get them off your mind.
- Read for relaxation before you fall asleep or take a warm bath.

—James B. Maas, PhD
Professor of Psychology, Cornell University
Author, *Power Sleep*

Date _____ Deep Breathing _____ Sleep _____
HOURS

Water ⬜ ⬜ ⬜ ⬜ ⬜ ⬜ ⬜ ⬜   Blood Pressure _____

F O O D

BREAKFAST   Time _____ Total Carb_____

　　　　　Serving Size   Food and Drinks

Grain
Vegetable
Protein
Fruit
Milk
Fat

SNACK   Time _____ Total Carb_____

LUNCH   Time _____ Total Carb_____

　　　　　Serving Size   Food and Drinks

Grain
Vegetable
Protein
Fruit
Milk
Fat

SNACK   Time _____ Total Carb_____

DINNER   Time _____ Total Carb_____

　　　　　Serving Size   Food and Drinks

Grain
Vegetable
Protein
Fruit
Milk
Fat

TOTALS

VEGETABLES   FRUIT   NUTS   WHOLE GRAINS

FUN	EMOTIONS	MOOD	ILLNESS	STRESS

Energy Level 1 2 3 4 5 6 7 8 9 10

MOVEMENT

Time of Day   Comments

Walking _____ steps/minutes

Weights _____ lbs, _____ reps

Stretches _____ minutes

Laughter _____

Other _____   **Weight** _____

BLOOD GLUCOSE NUMBERS

Time	Breakfast		Lunch		Dinner		Bedtime
	Before	After	Before	After	Before	After	

MEDICATIONS

Time	Type

Pillow Talk

Power naps do the job:

- 38% of the workforce nap on the job every week, often in their car or bathroom stall; the best is to put your head down for a 15–20-minute power nap.
- 27% of North Americans fall asleep at the wheel each year; best advice is to pull off the road and take a 15–20-minute power nap! Coffee and cool air won't help!
- Power naps are never more than 20 minutes, otherwise you feel even more tired.

Avoiding jet lag when you travel:

- Set your clock to destination time and start living at that time schedule.
- Avoid alcohol and heavy meals on the plane.
- Going East—if you land early, get out in the daylight and reset your body clock.
- Going West—stay up later in the day.
- Don't take a power nap when you arrive, that will keep you on your local time.

—James B. Maas, PhD
Professor of Psychology, Cornell University
Author, *Power Sleep*

Date _____ Deep Breathing _____ Sleep _____
HOURS

Water ▯ ▯ ▯ ▯ ▯ ▯ ▯ ▯   Blood Pressure _____

F O O D

BREAKFAST   Time _____ Total Carb_____

	Serving Size	Food and Drinks
Grain		
Vegetable		
Protein		
Fruit		
Milk		
Fat		

SNACK   Time _____ Total Carb_____

LUNCH   Time _____ Total Carb_____

	Serving Size	Food and Drinks
Grain		
Vegetable		
Protein		
Fruit		
Milk		
Fat		

SNACK   Time _____ Total Carb_____

DINNER   Time _____ Total Carb_____

	Serving Size	Food and Drinks
Grain		
Vegetable		
Protein		
Fruit		
Milk		
Fat		

TOTALS

VEGETABLES   FRUIT   NUTS   WHOLE GRAINS

FUN	EMOTIONS	MOOD	ILLNESS	STRESS

Energy Level 1 2 3 4 5 6 7 8 9 10

MOVEMENT

Time of Day   Comments

Walking _____ steps/minutes

Weights _____ lbs, _____ reps

Stretches _____ minutes

Laughter _____

Other _____   **Weight** _____

BLOOD GLUCOSE NUMBERS

Time	Breakfast		Lunch		Dinner		Bedtime
	Before	After	Before	After	Before	After	

MEDICATIONS

Time	Type

Sustainable Food Systems for Better Health and Enhanced Environment

We must be able to grow food to eat without damaging the environment and endangering future generations. There is more to consider than the crop in the ground at this moment. The qualities of real food are: health (contains vitamins, minerals, and fiber), nature (easy on the planet), joy (bringing people back to the table to celebrate life together), and justice (sustains people for centuries). Rice and beans are examples of foods that have been cultivated for centuries and continue to prove to be healthy for us to eat.

- Real foods are often organic or ethnic foods.
- Real food should be part of programs giving food to those who cannot afford it.
- Real food measures suggest using meat as a garnish and purchasing more plant foods.

—Rod MacRae, PhD
Director, Food Policy Council

For further information on this topic contact: www.realfoodhome.net

Date _____ Deep Breathing _____ Sleep _____
HOURS

Water ⬜ ⬜ ⬜ ⬜ ⬜ ⬜ ⬜ ⬜   Blood Pressure _____

FOOD

BREAKFAST   Time _____ Total Carb_____

	Serving Size	Food and Drinks
Grain		
Vegetable		
Protein		
Fruit		
Milk		
Fat		

SNACK   Time _____ Total Carb_____

LUNCH   Time _____ Total Carb_____

	Serving Size	Food and Drinks
Grain		
Vegetable		
Protein		
Fruit		
Milk		
Fat		

SNACK   Time _____ Total Carb_____

DINNER   Time _____ Total Carb_____

	Serving Size	Food and Drinks
Grain		
Vegetable		
Protein		
Fruit		
Milk		
Fat		

TOTALS

VEGETABLES   FRUIT   NUTS   WHOLE GRAINS

FUN	EMOTIONS	MOOD	ILLNESS	STRESS

Energy Level 1 2 3 4 5 6 7 8 9 10

MOVEMENT

Time of Day   Comments

Walking _____ steps/minutes

Weights _____ lbs, _____ reps

Stretches _____ minutes

Laughter _____

Other _____

Weight _____

BLOOD GLUCOSE NUMBERS

Time	Breakfast		Lunch		Dinner		Bedtime
	Before	After	Before	After	Before	After	

MEDICATIONS

Time	Type

Healthy Insight for the Day

Ingredients for a healthy diet
- Fresh, natural, flavorful, and often locally grown ingredients.
- Moderate servings (just a teaspoon, especially if high in fat, is best).
- It's one of life's greatest pleasures.
- Focus on what you add to your diet for greater nutritional benefits.

Ingredients for a great recipe
- A recipe is only as good as the ingredients you use.
- Use fresh, wholesome, flavorful, natural ingredients for best health and flavor (Graham: Get to your food fast before someone gets to it first; the fresher the better!)
- Use high-fat ingredients in moderate amounts to make recipes tasty yet light. If it doesn't taste good, it won't be eaten, no matter what the nutritional benefits are.

—**Jill Melton, RD**
Senior Editor, *Cooking Light* Magazine

Date _____ Deep Breathing _____ Sleep _____

Water ⊔ ⊔ ⊔ ⊔ ⊔ ⊔ ⊔ ⊔   HOURS

Blood Pressure _____

F O O D

BREAKFAST

Time _____ Total Carb_____

	Serving Size	Food and Drinks
Grain		
Vegetable		
Protein		
Fruit		
Milk		
Fat		

SNACK

Time _____ Total Carb_____

LUNCH

Time _____ Total Carb_____

	Serving Size	Food and Drinks
Grain		
Vegetable		
Protein		
Fruit		
Milk		
Fat		

SNACK

Time _____ Total Carb_____

DINNER

Time _____ Total Carb_____

	Serving Size	Food and Drinks
Grain		
Vegetable		
Protein		
Fruit		
Milk		
Fat		

TOTALS

VEGETABLES   FRUIT   NUTS   WHOLE GRAINS

FUN	EMOTIONS	MOOD	ILLNESS	STRESS

Energy Level 1 2 3 4 5 6 7 8 9 10

MOVEMENT

Time of Day   Comments

Walking _____ steps/minutes

Weights _____ lbs, _____ reps

Stretches _____ minutes

Laughter _____

Other _____   **Weight** _____

BLOOD GLUCOSE NUMBERS

Time	Breakfast		Lunch		Dinner		Bedtime
	Before	After	Before	After	Before	After	

MEDICATIONS

Time	Type

Tips for the Traveler

- Eat simply and rely on natural and whole foods.
- Drinking bottled water and eating only fruit that you peel can help you avoid stomach upsets.
- Strive for balance between protein and carbohydrate.
- Be sure to get enough fiber in your meals and to drink enough water.
- Add orange juice to breakfast and be sure you are well hydrated throughout the day.
- Have a registered dietitian establish your meal guidelines so you can make requests ahead of time from the chef at the hotel and restaurants where you will eat.
- Request a healthy meal from the airlines; you can choose from several choices, including diabetic and vegetarian.

—**Jill Melton, RD**
Senior Editor, *Cooking Light* Magazine
www.cookinglight.com

Date _____ Deep Breathing _____ Sleep _____

Water ☐ ☐ ☐ ☐ ☐ ☐ ☐ ☐　　Blood Pressure _____

HOURS

F O O D

BREAKFAST
Time _____ Total Carb_____

	Serving Size	Food and Drinks
Grain		
Vegetable		
Protein		
Fruit		
Milk		
Fat		

SNACK
Time _____ Total Carb_____

LUNCH
Time _____ Total Carb_____

	Serving Size	Food and Drinks
Grain		
Vegetable		
Protein		
Fruit		
Milk		
Fat		

SNACK
Time _____ Total Carb_____

DINNER
Time _____ Total Carb_____

	Serving Size	Food and Drinks
Grain		
Vegetable		
Protein		
Fruit		
Milk		
Fat		

TOTALS

VEGETABLES　　　FRUIT　　　NUTS　　　WHOLE GRAINS

FUN	EMOTIONS	MOOD	ILLNESS	STRESS

Energy Level 1   2   3   4   5   6   7   8   9   10

MOVEMENT

Time of Day   Comments

Walking _____ steps/minutes

Weights _____ lbs, _____ reps

Stretches _____ minutes

Laughter _____

Other _____   **Weight** _____

BLOOD GLUCOSE NUMBERS

Time	Breakfast		Lunch		Dinner		Bedtime
	Before	After	Before	After	Before	After	

MEDICATIONS

Time	Type

How to Read the Research

Does it sound too good to be true?

What is the source of the information; who did it?

Does the research benefit a certain business?

After hearing about a great new pill, diet, or health fix, people buy it and often take too much because they think more is better. People become their own guinea pigs, and this results in a natural experiment that we hear about when something goes wrong. For example, B6 was touted for carpal tunnel syndrome, but taken in excess by itself, it caused nerve damage. To save money and possible health risk, avoid these pitfalls!

Remember that no single study can give us the whole story. Worthwhile research stands the test of time. Ask a health professional (doctor or a dietitian) to filter scientific evidence into practice for you when you have health-related questions.

—**Rena A. Mendelson, DSc, MS**
Associate VP Academics, Ryerson Polytechnic
University

Date _____ Deep Breathing _____ Sleep _____
HOURS

Water ▯ ▯ ▯ ▯ ▯ ▯ ▯ ▯ Blood Pressure _____

F O O D

BREAKFAST
Time _____ Total Carb_____

Serving Size   Food and Drinks

Grain
Vegetable
Protein
Fruit
Milk
Fat

SNACK
Time _____ Total Carb_____

LUNCH
Time _____ Total Carb_____

Serving Size   Food and Drinks

Grain
Vegetable
Protein
Fruit
Milk
Fat

SNACK
Time _____ Total Carb_____

DINNER
Time _____ Total Carb_____

Serving Size   Food and Drinks

Grain
Vegetable
Protein
Fruit
Milk
Fat

T O T A L S

VEGETABLES   FRUIT   NUTS   WHOLE GRAINS

FUN	EMOTIONS	MOOD	ILLNESS	STRESS

Energy Level 1 2 3 4 5 6 7 8 9 10

MOVEMENT

Time of Day   Comments

Walking _____ steps/minutes

Weights _____ lbs, _____ reps

Stretches _____ minutes

Laughter _____

Other _____   **Weight** _____

BLOOD GLUCOSE NUMBERS

Time	Breakfast Before	Breakfast After	Lunch Before	Lunch After	Dinner Before	Dinner After	Bedtime

MEDICATIONS

Time	Type

Saturated Fat

Saturated fat, not cholesterol, is the true culprit of the Western diet. It is found in coconut, shortening, bacon, red meats, butter, hard cheese, and whole milk. This type of fat makes our bodies produce more cholesterol, and this can lead to heart disease, so we should limit this type of fat. We can eat all foods and be healthy, but remember balance, variety and moderation! If you have butter, choose a small amount!

Food labels in the United States are standardized, so they list the same nutrients, such as saturated fat, carbohydrate, and fiber, allowing you to compare products to get the healthiest one. Read the ingredients that are in the food. The ingredient list tells all, including trans fats (hydrogenated vegetable oil) and chemical preservatives. If saturated fats are listed, you may want to eat a smaller serving of that food.

—Nelda Mercer, MS, RD
American Dietetic Association Spokesperson,
www.mfitnutrition.com

Date _____ Deep Breathing _____ Sleep _____

Water 🥛 🥛 🥛 🥛 🥛 🥛 🥛 🥛   Blood Pressure _____

HOURS

F O O D

BREAKFAST   Time _____ Total Carb_____

	Serving Size	Food and Drinks
Grain		
Vegetable		
Protein		
Fruit		
Milk		
Fat		

SNACK   Time _____ Total Carb_____

LUNCH   Time _____ Total Carb_____

	Serving Size	Food and Drinks
Grain		
Vegetable		
Protein		
Fruit		
Milk		
Fat		

SNACK   Time _____ Total Carb_____

DINNER   Time _____ Total Carb_____

	Serving Size	Food and Drinks
Grain		
Vegetable		
Protein		
Fruit		
Milk		
Fat		

TOTALS

VEGETABLES   FRUIT   NUTS   WHOLE GRAINS

FUN	EMOTIONS	MOOD	ILLNESS	STRESS

Energy Level   1   2   3   4   5   6   7   8   9   10

MOVEMENT

Time of Day   Comments

Walking _____ steps/minutes

Weights   _____ lbs, _____ reps

Stretches _____ minutes

Laughter _____

Other   _____   **Weight** _____

BLOOD GLUCOSE NUMBERS

Time	Breakfast		Lunch		Dinner		Bedtime
	Before	After	Before	After	Before	After	

MEDICATIONS

Time	Type

Healthy Insight for the Day

Today's customer is more affluent and eats out often—50% of the entire food budget is consumed away from home. Foods cannot be rich all of the time when people are eating out so often, but people want to eat well and feel good when they get up from the table.

People graze through the appetizer menu instead of ordering just one course. So, chefs must create a healthy cuisine and low-fat dishes that taste good.

The best quality ingredients yield the best end-result. Not a lot has to be done to make recipes taste great when there is great food to start with. Non-stick pans are of great help.

Fast cooking, grilling, and poaching are methods of cooking that accentuate aromas and flavors. "Good Nutrition is nothing more than good food, properly selected and carefully prepared. And nothing less."

—Ferdinand Metz, CMC
President, The Culinary Institute of America,
www.ciachef.edu

Date _____ Deep Breathing _____ Sleep _____
HOURS

Water ☐ ☐ ☐ ☐ ☐ ☐ ☐ ☐   Blood Pressure _____

F O O D

BREAKFAST   Time _____ Total Carb_____

      Serving Size   Food and Drinks
Grain
Vegetable
Protein
Fruit
Milk
Fat

SNACK   Time _____ Total Carb_____

LUNCH   Time _____ Total Carb_____

      Serving Size   Food and Drinks
Grain
Vegetable
Protein
Fruit
Milk
Fat

SNACK   Time _____ Total Carb_____

DINNER   Time _____ Total Carb_____

      Serving Size   Food and Drinks
Grain
Vegetable
Protein
Fruit
Milk
Fat

T O T A L S

VEGETABLES   FRUIT   NUTS   WHOLE GRAINS

FUN	EMOTIONS	MOOD	ILLNESS	STRESS

Energy Level 1 2 3 4 5 6 7 8 9 10

MOVEMENT

Time of Day   Comments

Walking _____ steps/minutes

Weights _____ lbs, _____ reps

Stretches _____ minutes

Laughter _____

Other _____   Weight _____

BLOOD GLUCOSE NUMBERS

Time	Breakfast		Lunch		Dinner		Bedtime
	Before	After	Before	After	Before	After	

MEDICATIONS

Time	Type

Exercise and Diabetes

Why is exercise so beneficial, especially to those with diabetes?

It helps to circulate insulin throughout the body in the blood supply.

With this better circulation, blood sugar gets into the cells more efficiently.

Blood sugar levels respond by coming down.

Exercise is a very important part of preventing diabetes or managing diabetes, once a person has it.

The power of exercise is that once you start exercising, you benefit 24 hours a day from a 20–30-minute workout.

—Cathy Mullooly, MS, CDE
Director of Physiology, Joslin Diabetes Center

Date _____ Deep Breathing _____ Sleep _____
HOURS

Water 🥛 🥛 🥛 🥛 🥛 🥛 🥛 🥛 Blood Pressure _____

F O O D

BREAKFAST   Time _____ Total Carb_____

          Serving Size   Food and Drinks
Grain
Vegetable
Protein
Fruit
Milk
Fat

SNACK   Time _____ Total Carb_____

LUNCH   Time _____ Total Carb_____

          Serving Size   Food and Drinks
Grain
Vegetable
Protein
Fruit
Milk
Fat

SNACK   Time _____ Total Carb_____

DINNER   Time _____ Total Carb_____

          Serving Size   Food and Drinks
Grain
Vegetable
Protein
Fruit
Milk
Fat

T O T A L S

VEGETABLES   FRUIT   NUTS   WHOLE GRAINS

Energy Level   1   2   3   4   5   6   7   8   9   10

MOVEMENT

Time of Day   Comments

Walking ——————— steps/minutes

Weights ——————— lbs, ——————— reps

Stretches ——————— minutes

Laughter ———————

Other ————————————————————   Weight ———————————

BLOOD GLUCOSE NUMBERS

Time	Breakfast		Lunch		Dinner		Bedtime
	Before	After	Before	After	Before	After	

MEDICATIONS

Time	Type

Can My Blood Sugar Go Too Low with Exercise?

If you take insulin or a sulfonylurea, your blood sugar might go too low.

- Check your blood glucose before you exercise, and if it is below 100, have a snack, such as half a meat sandwich. If you exercise for longer than an hour, check your blood sugar again. Check again 30 minutes after you finish exercising. Vigorous exercise can lower your blood sugar for up to 24 hours. Low blood sugar can make you feel extremely tired and confused. Always wear medical identification in case you have a low when you are away from home and need some help.
- Be prepared to treat a low by carrying with you glucose gel or tablets, peanut butter crackers, sports bars, sports drinks, raisins, hard candy, or juice.
- It is wise to time your exercise for after meals to meet the rise in blood sugar and bring it back down.

—Cathy Mullooly, MS, CDE
Director of Physiology, Joslin Diabetes Center

Date _____ Deep Breathing _____ Sleep _____
HOURS

Water ▢ ▢ ▢ ▢ ▢ ▢ ▢ ▢   Blood Pressure _____

F O O D

BREAKFAST   Time _____ Total Carb_____

　　　　Serving Size   Food and Drinks
Grain
Vegetable
Protein
Fruit
Milk
Fat

SNACK   Time _____ Total Carb_____

LUNCH   Time _____ Total Carb_____

　　　　Serving Size   Food and Drinks
Grain
Vegetable
Protein
Fruit
Milk
Fat

SNACK   Time _____ Total Carb_____

DINNER   Time _____ Total Carb_____

　　　　Serving Size   Food and Drinks
Grain
Vegetable
Protein
Fruit
Milk
Fat

TOTALS

VEGETABLES   FRUIT   NUTS   WHOLE GRAINS

FUN	EMOTIONS	MOOD	ILLNESS	STRESS

Energy Level   1   2   3   4   5   6   7   8   9   10

MOVEMENT

Time of Day   Comments

Walking _____ steps/minutes

Weights _____ lbs, _____ reps

Stretches _____ minutes

Laughter _____

Other _____   Weight _____

BLOOD GLUCOSE NUMBERS

Time	Breakfast		Lunch		Dinner		Bedtime
	Before	After	Before	After	Before	After	

MEDICATIONS

Time	Type

There is a Way

For people with feet or leg problems that want to keep on exercising:

- Stationary bicycle
- Pool exercise programs
- Rowing machines
- Arm and leg movements in a chair
- Seated yoga and stretches
- Seated weight-lifting using light weights or bags of rice
- Seated resistance exercises using bands or balls
- Tai chi

Meet with a qualified exercise physiologist before you begin an exercise program.

—Cathy Mullooly, MS, CDE
Director of Physiology, Joslin Diabetes Center

Date _____ Deep Breathing _____ Sleep _____

HOURS

Water ⬭ ⬭ ⬭ ⬭ ⬭ ⬭ ⬭ ⬭ Blood Pressure _____

F O O D

BREAKFAST   Time _____ Total Carb_____

    Serving Size   Food and Drinks

Grain
Vegetable
Protein
Fruit
Milk
Fat

SNACK   Time _____ Total Carb_____

LUNCH   Time _____ Total Carb_____

    Serving Size   Food and Drinks

Grain
Vegetable
Protein
Fruit
Milk
Fat

SNACK   Time _____ Total Carb_____

DINNER   Time _____ Total Carb_____

    Serving Size   Food and Drinks

Grain
Vegetable
Protein
Fruit
Milk
Fat

T O T A L S

VEGETABLES   FRUIT   NUTS   WHOLE GRAINS

FUN	EMOTIONS	MOOD	ILLNESS	STRESS

Energy Level 1 2 3 4 5 6 7 8 9 10

MOVEMENT

Time of Day   Comments

Walking _____ steps/minutes

Weights _____ lbs, _____ reps

Stretches _____ minutes

Laughter _____

Other _____   Weight _____

BLOOD GLUCOSE NUMBERS

Time	Breakfast		Lunch		Dinner		Bedtime
	Before	After	Before	After	Before	After	

MEDICATIONS

Time	Type

You're Never Too Old

It is never too late to start exercising; the older you are, the more important it is to be active!

The proven benefits of exercise in elders:
- Reduces CAD, blood pressure, and arthritis symptoms.
- Improves physical and mental well-being.
- Increases bone density, mobility, lung capacity, muscle mass and tone, strength, flexibility, and endurance.
- Helps seniors be independent in their day-to-day tasks—and make friends.

SilverSneakers offers seniors with certain health plans or insurance full membership in many fitness facilities in their area, free of charge. For information go to www.silversneakers.com or call 800-295-4993. If SilverSneakers is not in your area, your physician and an exercise physiologist can help you with an exercise plan.

—Steve Nelson, MBA
Former Senior VP, Healthcare Dimensions

Date _____ Deep Breathing _____ Sleep _____
HOURS

Water ☐ ☐ ☐ ☐ ☐ ☐ ☐ ☐   Blood Pressure _____

F O O D

BREAKFAST   Time _____ Total Carb_____

        Serving Size   Food and Drinks

Grain
Vegetable
Protein
Fruit
Milk
Fat

SNACK   Time _____ Total Carb_____

LUNCH   Time _____ Total Carb_____

        Serving Size   Food and Drinks

Grain
Vegetable
Protein
Fruit
Milk
Fat

SNACK   Time _____ Total Carb_____

DINNER   Time _____ Total Carb_____

        Serving Size   Food and Drinks

Grain
Vegetable
Protein
Fruit
Milk
Fat

T O T A L S

VEGETABLES   FRUIT   NUTS   WHOLE GRAINS

Energy Level 1 2 3 4 5 6 7 8 9 10

MOVEMENT

Time of Day   Comments

Walking _____ steps/minutes

Weights _____ lbs, _____ reps

Stretches _____ minutes

Laughter _____

Other _____ Weight _____

BLOOD GLUCOSE NUMBERS

Time	Breakfast		Lunch		Dinner		Bedtime
	Before	After	Before	After	Before	After	

MEDICATIONS

Time	Type

How Simple Is a Healthy Diet?

Two changes in the typical adult diet will help:
- Balancing calories through more activity and eating less food overall.
- Focus on eating more fruits and vegetables, as the best move toward a more balanced and healthy diet. A disease-fighting diet has lots of fruits, vegetables, and whole grains; a moderate amount of milk, meat, and dairy products; and only little bits of fat, salt, and sugar.
- Don't overeat; cut servings in half.
- Exercise gives you enormous benefits, even just with walking 1 mile a day, so you don't have to run a marathon, or even run!
- When making lifelong changes in your diet and lifestyle, a partial commitment is okay. Don't feel you have to do it all at once, and don't set unrealistic goals.

—**Marion Nestle, PhD, MPH**
Chair, Nutrition & Food Studies, New York University
www.nyu.edu/education/nutrition

Date _____ Deep Breathing _____ Sleep _____
                                                                        HOURS
Water ☐ ☐ ☐ ☐ ☐ ☐ ☐ ☐   Blood Pressure _____

F O O D

BREAKFAST   Time _____ Total Carb_____

     Serving Size   Food and Drinks
Grain
Vegetable
Protein
Fruit
Milk
Fat

SNACK   Time _____ Total Carb_____

LUNCH   Time _____ Total Carb_____

     Serving Size   Food and Drinks
Grain
Vegetable
Protein
Fruit
Milk
Fat

SNACK   Time _____ Total Carb_____

DINNER   Time _____ Total Carb_____

     Serving Size   Food and Drinks
Grain
Vegetable
Protein
Fruit
Milk
Fat

T O T A L S

VEGETABLES   FRUIT   NUTS   WHOLE GRAINS

FUN	EMOTIONS	MOOD	ILLNESS	STRESS

Energy Level 1 2 3 4 5 6 7 8 9 10

MOVEMENT

Time of Day   Comments

Walking _____ steps/minutes

Weights   _____ lbs, _____ reps

Stretches   _____ minutes

Laughter   _____

Other   _____   **Weight** _____

BLOOD GLUCOSE NUMBERS

Time	Breakfast		Lunch		Dinner		Bedtime
	Before	After	Before	After	Before	After	

MEDICATIONS

Time	Type

Healthy Insight for the Day

We live in the era of super-size and all-you-can-eat deals, when we rarely need more than half the portion that is served. The bigger the portion, the more calories you end up consuming! To keep your calories in check:

- Cut a portion in half.
- Don't buy the largest item, no matter how good the deal is.
- Share your meal with someone else.

What's the problem with the fat-free craze?
People think that if a food is labeled fat free, they can eat as much as they want. Nope, it may be fat free, but it is not calorie free. Fat-free products usually have more sugar or carbohydrate to make up for the change in texture and taste. Fat-free mania has resulted in people eating too much, leading to weight gain. We don't suggest you eat "no fat" foods, but smaller amounts of healthy fats for your health.

—Marion Nestle, PhD, MPH
Chair, Nutrition & Food Studies, New York University
www.nyu.edu/education/nutrition

Date _____ Deep Breathing _____ Sleep _____
HOURS

Water ☐ ☐ ☐ ☐ ☐ ☐ ☐ ☐　　Blood Pressure _____

F O O D

BREAKFAST　　　　　　Time _____ Total Carb_____

　　　　Serving Size　　Food and Drinks

Grain
Vegetable
Protein
Fruit
Milk
Fat

SNACK　　　　　　　　Time _____ Total Carb_____

LUNCH　　　　　　　　Time _____ Total Carb_____

　　　　Serving Size　　Food and Drinks

Grain
Vegetable
Protein
Fruit
Milk
Fat

SNACK　　　　　　　　Time _____ Total Carb_____

DINNER　　　　　　　Time _____ Total Carb_____

　　　　Serving Size　　Food and Drinks

Grain
Vegetable
Protein
Fruit
Milk
Fat

T O T A L S

VEGETABLES　　　　FRUIT　　　　NUTS　　　　WHOLE GRAINS

FUN	EMOTIONS	MOOD	ILLNESS	STRESS

Energy Level 1 2 3 4 5 6 7 8 9 10

MOVEMENT

Time of Day   Comments

Walking _____ steps/minutes

Weights _____ lbs, _____ reps

Stretches _____ minutes

Laughter _____

Other _____   **Weight** _____

BLOOD GLUCOSE NUMBERS

Time	Breakfast		Lunch		Dinner		Bedtime
	Before	After	Before	After	Before	After	

MEDICATIONS

Time	Type

Our Food Supply

It is possible to eat a fabulous diet from supermarket foods. Our food supply is abundant with healthy choices at reasonable prices, and if you eat a variety of foods in a balanced way, you will be well nourished and reduce your disease risk.

Strive for fresh fruits, vegetables, whole grains and beans as the focus of your diet. Keep dairy and meat servings small, and the smallest of all are added fats and sugars. It is up to you to change the environment around you to one that is encouraging to healthier living. Walk more, eat less, and most of all, enjoy food for the great pleasure that it can give to us all.

—Marion Nestle, PhD, MPH
Chair, Nutrition & Food Studies, New York University
www.nyu.edu/education/nutrition

Date _____ Deep Breathing _____ Sleep _____
HOURS

Water ▯ ▯ ▯ ▯ ▯ ▯ ▯ ▯   Blood Pressure _____

F O O D

BREAKFAST   Time _____ Total Carb_____

	Serving Size	Food and Drinks
Grain		
Vegetable		
Protein		
Fruit		
Milk		
Fat		

SNACK   Time _____ Total Carb_____

LUNCH   Time _____ Total Carb_____

	Serving Size	Food and Drinks
Grain		
Vegetable		
Protein		
Fruit		
Milk		
Fat		

SNACK   Time _____ Total Carb_____

DINNER   Time _____ Total Carb_____

	Serving Size	Food and Drinks
Grain		
Vegetable		
Protein		
Fruit		
Milk		
Fat		

TOTALS

VEGETABLES   FRUIT   NUTS   WHOLE GRAINS

FUN	EMOTIONS	MOOD	ILLNESS	STRESS

Energy Level   1   2   3   4   5   6   7   8   9   10

MOVEMENT

                  Time of Day   Comments

Walking _____ steps/minutes

Weights _____ lbs, _____ reps

Stretches _____ minutes

Laughter _____

Other _____   **Weight** _____

BLOOD GLUCOSE NUMBERS

Time	Breakfast		Lunch		Dinner		Bedtime
	Before	After	Before	After	Before	After	

MEDICATIONS

Time	Type

Going All the Way with Organics

We only use organic foods in our restaurants, because it tastes great, and it's better for you.

You can find organic food at:

- Farmers' markets
- Organic distributors
- Health food stores, such as Whole Foods Market
- Local supermarkets, such as Safeway and Giant
- Community supported agriculture co-ops

Agricultural centers at universities often know about local farmers' markets and community supported agriculture, which is a way to get the very freshest produce outside of your own garden.

—Nora Pouillon
Chef/Owner, Restaurant Nora and Asia Nora

For further information go to: www.noras.com

Date _____ Deep Breathing _____ Sleep _____
HOURS

Water ⬜ ⬜ ⬜ ⬜ ⬜ ⬜ ⬜ ⬜   Blood Pressure _____

F O O D

BREAKFAST   Time _____ Total Carb_____

    Serving Size   Food and Drinks

Grain
Vegetable
Protein
Fruit
Milk
Fat

SNACK   Time _____ Total Carb_____

LUNCH   Time _____ Total Carb_____

    Serving Size   Food and Drinks

Grain
Vegetable
Protein
Fruit
Milk
Fat

SNACK   Time _____ Total Carb_____

DINNER   Time _____ Total Carb_____

    Serving Size   Food and Drinks

Grain
Vegetable
Protein
Fruit
Milk
Fat

TOTALS

VEGETABLES   FRUIT   NUTS   WHOLE GRAINS

Energy Level   1   2   3   4   5   6   7   8   9   10

MOVEMENT

Time of Day   Comments

Walking _____ steps/minutes

Weights _____ lbs, _____ reps

Stretches _____ minutes

Laughter _____

Other _____   Weight _____

BLOOD GLUCOSE NUMBERS							
	Breakfast		Lunch		Dinner		
Time	Before	After	Before	After	Before	After	Bedtime

MEDICATIONS	
Time	Type

GRAHAM

Each person should be able to identify the stage of change he is in. With awareness and help from professionals, each of us can move through the stages of change and succeed with our health behavior goals.

The Five Stages of Change

Precontemplation: not ready to change, may have given up on ability to change*

Contemplation: thinking about change, but have real doubts*

Preparation: taking small steps to get ready to change, making a plan

Action: making a visible change (for less than six months)

Maintenance: continuing for more than six months, be prepared for backsliding so you don't return to old habits

*Often the hardest part is moving from precontemplation to contemplation, because people don't know the many benefits of making change (healthier heart, healthier brain, sleep better).

—James Prochaska, PhD
Author, *Changing For Good*

Date _____ Deep Breathing _____ Sleep _____
HOURS

Water ⬜ ⬜ ⬜ ⬜ ⬜ ⬜ ⬜ ⬜   Blood Pressure _____

F O O D

BREAKFAST   Time _____ Total Carb_____

      Serving Size   Food and Drinks

Grain
Vegetable
Protein
Fruit
Milk
Fat

SNACK   Time _____ Total Carb_____

LUNCH   Time _____ Total Carb_____

      Serving Size   Food and Drinks

Grain
Vegetable
Protein
Fruit
Milk
Fat

SNACK   Time _____ Total Carb_____

DINNER   Time _____ Total Carb_____

      Serving Size   Food and Drinks

Grain
Vegetable
Protein
Fruit
Milk
Fat

TOTALS

VEGETABLES   FRUIT   NUTS   WHOLE GRAINS

FUN	EMOTIONS	MOOD	ILLNESS	STRESS

Energy Level 1 2 3 4 5 6 7 8 9 10

MOVEMENT

Time of Day   Comments

Walking _____ steps/minutes

Weights _____ lbs, _____ reps

Stretches _____ minutes

Laughter _____

Other _____

Weight _____

BLOOD GLUCOSE NUMBERS

Time	Breakfast		Lunch		Dinner		Bedtime
	Before	After	Before	After	Before	After	

MEDICATIONS

Time	Type

Never Give Up Changing

To make a change transparent and just part of your routine, it may take 7–10 years on your own or close to 12 months with the correct guidance, and you may experience relapse along the way.

Backsliding or Relapse

Used to be, relapse was considered failure, but it's really a learning experience.

Ask yourself "Why did I backslide? Did I make a mistake? What will I do differently next time I make a mistake?"

The only true mistake is to give up on yourself and your ability to change.

—**James Prochaska, PhD**
Director, Cancer Prevention Research Center,
Professor of Psychology, University of Rhode Island
Author, *Changing For Good*

For more information contact: www.prochange.com

Date _____ Deep Breathing _____ Sleep _____
HOURS

Water ☐ ☐ ☐ ☐ ☐ ☐ ☐ ☐   Blood Pressure _____

F O O D

BREAKFAST   Time _____ Total Carb_____

       Serving Size   Food and Drinks

Grain
Vegetable
Protein
Fruit
Milk
Fat

SNACK   Time _____ Total Carb_____

LUNCH   Time _____ Total Carb_____

       Serving Size   Food and Drinks

Grain
Vegetable
Protein
Fruit
Milk
Fat

SNACK   Time _____ Total Carb_____

DINNER   Time _____ Total Carb_____

       Serving Size   Food and Drinks

Grain
Vegetable
Protein
Fruit
Milk
Fat

T O T A L S

VEGETABLES   FRUIT   NUTS   WHOLE GRAINS

FUN	EMOTIONS	MOOD	ILLNESS	STRESS

Energy Level 1   2   3   4   5   6   7   8   9   10

MOVEMENT

Time of Day   Comments

Walking _____ steps/minutes

Weights _____ lbs, _____ reps

Stretches _____ minutes

Laughter _____

Other _____   **Weight** _____

BLOOD GLUCOSE NUMBERS

Time	Breakfast		Lunch		Dinner		Bedtime
	Before	After	Before	After	Before	After	

MEDICATIONS

Time	Type

Low-Fat Baking

Eggs: (be careful because egg whites tend to dry out cake batter)

- 2 whole eggs = 2 egg whites and leave out the yolks or 3 whites, but not more
- 3 eggs = 1 whole egg and 2 whites

Fat: For each cup of fat in a recipe, try these suggestions:

- Take out 1/4 cup of fat automatically, you will get just a slightly different texture.
- Try 1/3 or 1/4 cup puree (applesauce, baby food, apricot, or pear puree).
- Try 1/4 or 1/3 cup canola or light olive oil.
- Try 1/4 cup yogurt, which adds flavor and moisture and has acidity that tenderizes the gluten in the flour for a tender product.
- Use corn syrup (dark and light), which is viscous, holds air and moisture, and gives flavor and some tenderizing.
- Key for all high-fat ingredients: Don't cut it out, but cut back!

—Susan Purdy
Award Winning Cookbook Author
Have Your Cake and Eat It, Too
and *Let Them Eat Cake*

Date _____ Deep Breathing _____ Sleep _____
HOURS

Water ⬜ ⬜ ⬜ ⬜ ⬜ ⬜ ⬜ ⬜   Blood Pressure _____

F O O D

BREAKFAST   Time _____   Total Carb_____

     Serving Size   Food and Drinks

Grain
Vegetable
Protein
Fruit
Milk
Fat

SNACK   Time _____   Total Carb_____

LUNCH   Time _____   Total Carb_____

     Serving Size   Food and Drinks

Grain
Vegetable
Protein
Fruit
Milk
Fat

SNACK   Time _____   Total Carb_____

DINNER   Time _____   Total Carb_____

     Serving Size   Food and Drinks

Grain
Vegetable
Protein
Fruit
Milk
Fat

T O T A L S

VEGETABLES   FRUIT   NUTS   WHOLE GRAINS

FUN	EMOTIONS	MOOD	ILLNESS	STRESS

Energy Level 1 2 3 4 5 6 7 8 9 10

MOVEMENT

Time of Day   Comments

Walking _____ steps/minutes

Weights _____ lbs, _____ reps

Stretches _____ minutes

Laughter _____

Other _____   **Weight** _____

BLOOD GLUCOSE NUMBERS

Time	Breakfast		Lunch		Dinner		Bedtime
	Before	After	Before	After	Before	After	

MEDICATIONS

Time	Type

Low-Fat Baking

Flour:
- Cake flour is milled from soft wheat that contains less protein, so you need less fat to tenderize the cake.
- Cornstarch can add tenderness.

More Low-Fat Baking Tips:
- To test doneness of a cake, test with a clean toothpick—there should be no "stickies."
- Place the baked cake on a trivet/rack so that the air circulates underneath and the condensation does not make the cake stick to the pan. Steam will settle out of the cake.
- Line the cake pan with a spritz of cooking spray, wax paper, and flour so the cake releases easily after being cooked.
- Use cocoa instead of flour when preparing a pan for a chocolate cake.

—Susan Purdy
Award Winning Cookbook Author
Have Your Cake and Eat It, Too
and *Let Them Eat Cake*

Date _____ Deep Breathing _____ Sleep _____
                                                                    HOURS
Water ⊔ ⊔ ⊔ ⊔ ⊔ ⊔ ⊔ ⊔   Blood Pressure _____

F O O D

BREAKFAST   Time _____ Total Carb_____

	Serving Size	Food and Drinks
Grain		
Vegetable		
Protein		
Fruit		
Milk		
Fat		

SNACK   Time _____ Total Carb_____

LUNCH   Time _____ Total Carb_____

	Serving Size	Food and Drinks
Grain		
Vegetable		
Protein		
Fruit		
Milk		
Fat		

SNACK   Time _____ Total Carb_____

DINNER   Time _____ Total Carb_____

	Serving Size	Food and Drinks
Grain		
Vegetable		
Protein		
Fruit		
Milk		
Fat		

T O T A L S

VEGETABLES   FRUIT   NUTS   WHOLE GRAINS

FUN	EMOTIONS	MOOD	ILLNESS	STRESS

Energy Level 1 2 3 4 5 6 7 8 9 10

MOVEMENT

Time of Day   Comments

Walking _____ steps/minutes

Weights _____ lbs, _____ reps

Stretches _____ minutes

Laughter _____

Other _____   **Weight** _____

BLOOD GLUCOSE NUMBERS

Time	Breakfast		Lunch		Dinner		Bedtime
	Before	After	Before	After	Before	After	

MEDICATIONS

Time	Type

Phytochemicals and Antioxidants

Phytochemicals: *Phyto* is derived from the ancient Greek word for plants. They are the compounds within plants that have the capacity for reaction and interaction. A single fruit or vegetable can contain thousands of phytochemicals in trace amounts, and they work synergistically with other phytochemicals. These unique substances can protect against heart disease, cancer, and other chronic diseases.

Antioxidants: Fight against oxygen products that can be damaging to the body (pollution, normal body processes) and protect cells; also found in fruits and vegetables.

Get more fruits and vegetables into your day, because it is important to eat foods, not supplements, to obtain the true benefits. The darker the colors of your fruit and vegetable choices, the more nutrients, phytochemicals, antioxidants, and fiber they contain.

—Regina Ragone, MS, RD
Food Editor, *Prevention* Magazine

Date _____ Deep Breathing _____ Sleep _____
HOURS

Water ☐ ☐ ☐ ☐ ☐ ☐ ☐ ☐   Blood Pressure _____

F O O D

BREAKFAST   Time _____ Total Carb_____

	Serving Size	Food and Drinks
Grain		
Vegetable		
Protein		
Fruit		
Milk		
Fat		

SNACK   Time _____ Total Carb_____

LUNCH   Time _____ Total Carb_____

	Serving Size	Food and Drinks
Grain		
Vegetable		
Protein		
Fruit		
Milk		
Fat		

SNACK   Time _____ Total Carb_____

DINNER   Time _____ Total Carb_____

	Serving Size	Food and Drinks
Grain		
Vegetable		
Protein		
Fruit		
Milk		
Fat		

TOTALS

VEGETABLES   FRUIT   NUTS   WHOLE GRAINS

FUN	EMOTIONS	MOOD	ILLNESS	STRESS

Energy Level 1 2 3 4 5 6 7 8 9 10

MOVEMENT

Time of Day   Comments

Walking _____ steps/minutes

Weights _____ lbs, _____ reps

Stretches _____ minutes

Laughter _____

Other _____   **Weight** _____

BLOOD GLUCOSE NUMBERS

Time	Breakfast Before	Breakfast After	Lunch Before	Lunch After	Dinner Before	Dinner After	Bedtime

MEDICATIONS

Time	Type

Here Are Five Phytochemicals Up Close

1. Allyl Sulfide in onion, garlic, and shallots lowers cholesterol, protects against cancer, and has antibacterial powers.

2. Beta-Carotene in orange-colored food like cantaloupe, squash, papaya, sweet potato, and carrots protect against cancers; it's a powerful antioxidant.

3. Lycopene, an antioxidant found in tomatos, protects against prostate cancer; best absorbed when tomatoes are cooked with a touch of fat (oil).

4. Quercetin, in onions, apples, and tea, may protect against cancer by blocking carcinogens and slow the growth and spread of cancer cells.

5. Genistein, in soy products like tempeh, soy milk, and tofu, is converted in the intestine to a compound that acts as a weak estrogen and can protect from hormone-related cancers such as breast cancer.

—Regina Ragone, MS, RD
Food Editor, *Prevention* Magazine

For more information contact: www.rodale.com

Date _____ Deep Breathing _____ Sleep _____
HOURS

Water ⬜ ⬜ ⬜ ⬜ ⬜ ⬜ ⬜ ⬜ Blood Pressure _____

F O O D

BREAKFAST
Time _____ Total Carb_____

      Serving Size   Food and Drinks

Grain
Vegetable
Protein
Fruit
Milk
Fat

SNACK
Time _____ Total Carb_____

LUNCH
Time _____ Total Carb_____

      Serving Size   Food and Drinks

Grain
Vegetable
Protein
Fruit
Milk
Fat

SNACK
Time _____ Total Carb_____

DINNER
Time _____ Total Carb_____

      Serving Size   Food and Drinks

Grain
Vegetable
Protein
Fruit
Milk
Fat

TOTALS

VEGETABLES   FRUIT   NUTS   WHOLE GRAINS

FUN	EMOTIONS	MOOD	ILLNESS	STRESS

Energy Level   1   2   3   4   5   6   7   8   9   10

MOVEMENT

Time of Day   Comments

Walking _____ steps/minutes

Weights _____ lbs, _____ reps

Stretches _____ minutes

Laughter _____

Other _____   **Weight** _____

BLOOD GLUCOSE NUMBERS

Time	Breakfast		Lunch		Dinner		Bedtime
	Before	After	Before	After	Before	After	

MEDICATIONS

Time	Type

Here Are Five More Phytochemicals Up Close

6. Indoles, in cruciferous vegetables like broccoli, cauliflower, Brussels sprouts, and cabbage, helps prevent carcinogens from reaching their target sites.

7. Sulforaphane, in cruciferous vegetables, especially broccoli, trigger an enzyme that transports carcinogens out of cells, bolstering the body's natural cancer-fighting ability.

8. Ellagic acid, in berries like strawberries, raspberries, and blueberries can ward off cancer.

9. Resveratrol, in wines, grapes, and peanuts, protects against heart disease.

10. Monoterpenes, in citrus fruit, cherries, spearmint, and dill are part of a large group that may prevent, slow, or reverse some cancers, and affect blood clotting and cholesterol.

—Regina Ragone, MS, RD
Food Editor, *Prevention* Magazine

For more information contact: www.rodale.com

Date _____ Deep Breathing _____ Sleep _____

HOURS

Water ⬜ ⬜ ⬜ ⬜ ⬜ ⬜ ⬜ ⬜   Blood Pressure _____

F O O D

BREAKFAST

Time _____ Total Carb_____

	Serving Size	Food and Drinks
Grain		
Vegetable		
Protein		
Fruit		
Milk		
Fat		

SNACK

Time _____ Total Carb_____

LUNCH

Time _____ Total Carb_____

	Serving Size	Food and Drinks
Grain		
Vegetable		
Protein		
Fruit		
Milk		
Fat		

SNACK

Time _____ Total Carb_____

DINNER

Time _____ Total Carb_____

	Serving Size	Food and Drinks
Grain		
Vegetable		
Protein		
Fruit		
Milk		
Fat		

TOTALS

VEGETABLES   FRUIT   NUTS   WHOLE GRAINS

FUN	EMOTIONS	MOOD	ILLNESS	STRESS

Energy Level   1   2   3   4   5   6   7   8   9   10

MOVEMENT

Time of Day   Comments

Walking _____ steps/minutes

Weights   _____ lbs, _____ reps

Stretches _____ minutes

Laughter   _____

Other   _____   **Weight** _____

BLOOD GLUCOSE NUMBERS

Time	Breakfast		Lunch		Dinner		Bedtime
	Before	After	Before	After	Before	After	

MEDICATIONS

Time	Type

Restaurant Savvy

Did you know a typical restaurant meal has 3,000 calories? (20% carbs, 40% protein, 40% fat)? Could you choose 1,000 calories (60% good carbs, 15% protein, and 25% fat)?

A reasonable portion of meat is 4 oz and of fish is 6 oz. Small meat portions go against our culture, but think of meat as an accompaniment to a meal rather than the main focus. Vegetables, whole grains, and legumes lend so much health to the diet that they should be the stars of the meal.

In buffets and cafeterias, you have control over the size of your servings, but in most restaurants, you don't. Try not to clean your plate. Instead, take home leftover portions or split meals with a friend. Talk to waiters and ask them to halve larger portions or if you can have a child's portion or an appetizer-sized serving. Take the initiative for the portions you want!

—**L. Timothy Ryan, CMC,**
Senior VP, The Culinary Institute of America,
www.ciachef.edu

Date _____ Deep Breathing _____ Sleep _____
HOURS

Water ☐ ☐ ☐ ☐ ☐ ☐ ☐ ☐   Blood Pressure _____

FOOD

BREAKFAST   Time _____ Total Carb_____

       Serving Size   Food and Drinks
Grain
Vegetable
Protein
Fruit
Milk
Fat

SNACK   Time _____ Total Carb_____

LUNCH   Time _____ Total Carb_____

       Serving Size   Food and Drinks
Grain
Vegetable
Protein
Fruit
Milk
Fat

SNACK   Time _____ Total Carb_____

DINNER   Time _____ Total Carb_____

       Serving Size   Food and Drinks
Grain
Vegetable
Protein
Fruit
Milk
Fat

TOTALS

VEGETABLES   FRUIT   NUTS   WHOLE GRAINS

FUN	EMOTIONS	MOOD	ILLNESS	STRESS

Energy Level   1   2   3   4   5   6   7   8   9   10

MOVEMENT

Time of Day   Comments

Walking _____ steps/minutes

Weights _____ lbs, _____ reps

Stretches _____ minutes

Laughter _____

Other _____   **Weight** _____

BLOOD GLUCOSE NUMBERS

Time	Breakfast		Lunch		Dinner		Bedtime
	Before	After	Before	After	Before	After	

MEDICATIONS

Time	Type

Can You Reverse Heart Disease?

(Well, Treena and I have made a good run at it, so we can honestly say yes.)

Heart disease is caused by injury to small arteries that feed your heart. Smoking, high blood pressure, sedentary lifestyle, and diabetes contribute to it. Genetics, diet, and high cholesterol affect heart disease, too.

- Limit saturated fat: dairy, meats, and baked goods are the main sources of saturated fat. The average person eats 50–75 grams of saturated fat daily.
- Reducing saturated fat to 15–20 grams dramatically reduces your cholesterol level and starts to reverse heart disease.
- Begin a walking program.
- Lower cholesterol levels to avoid heart surgery or angioplasty.
- Statin drugs can reduce risk of a second heart attack by 50%; make lifestyle changes, too.

—John Schroeder, MD
Professor, Cardiovascular Medicine,
Stanford University

Date _____ Deep Breathing _____ Sleep _____
                                                                      HOURS
Water ⬜ ⬜ ⬜ ⬜ ⬜ ⬜ ⬜ ⬜ Blood Pressure _____

F O O D

BREAKFAST   Time _____ Total Carb_____

    Serving Size   Food and Drinks
Grain
Vegetable
Protein
Fruit
Milk
Fat

SNACK   Time _____ Total Carb_____

LUNCH   Time _____ Total Carb_____

    Serving Size   Food and Drinks
Grain
Vegetable
Protein
Fruit
Milk
Fat

SNACK   Time _____ Total Carb_____

DINNER   Time _____ Total Carb_____

    Serving Size   Food and Drinks
Grain
Vegetable
Protein
Fruit
Milk
Fat

T O T A L S

VEGETABLES   FRUIT   NUTS   WHOLE GRAINS

FUN	EMOTIONS	MOOD	ILLNESS	STRESS

Energy Level   1   2   3   4   5   6   7   8   9   10

MOVEMENT

Time of Day   Comments

Walking _____ steps/minutes

Weights _____ lbs, _____ reps

Stretches _____ minutes

Laughter _____

Other _____

Weight _____

BLOOD GLUCOSE NUMBERS

Time	Breakfast		Lunch		Dinner		Bedtime
	Before	After	Before	After	Before	After	

MEDICATIONS

Time	Type

Know Your Numbers

Know your Numbers—then you can reverse your numbers!

If you have a family history of diabetes, stay thin, and exercise, which can delay or prevent this disease. Check blood sugar levels yearly, and if you have diabetes, take your medication and try lifestyle changes like a meal plan and daily walk to manage your blood sugar levels.

Keep total cholesterol under 200 mg/dl, LDL cholesterol less than 100mg/dl. If you cannot do it with lifestyle alone, see your doctor for medication, which may help.

If you have heart disease, diabetes, or high blood pressure, which are major risks for your heart, you may need to aim for a cholesterol value of 180mg/dl or lower.

—**John Schroeder, MD**
Professor, Cardiovascular Medicine,
Stanford University

For more information http://www.stanfordlifeplan.com/

Date _____ Deep Breathing _____ Sleep _____

HOURS

Water ☐ ☐ ☐ ☐ ☐ ☐ ☐ ☐   Blood Pressure _____

F O O D

BREAKFAST   Time _____ Total Carb_____

    Serving Size   Food and Drinks

Grain
Vegetable
Protein
Fruit
Milk
Fat

SNACK   Time _____ Total Carb_____

LUNCH   Time _____ Total Carb_____

    Serving Size   Food and Drinks

Grain
Vegetable
Protein
Fruit
Milk
Fat

SNACK   Time _____ Total Carb_____

DINNER   Time _____ Total Carb_____

    Serving Size   Food and Drinks

Grain
Vegetable
Protein
Fruit
Milk
Fat

T O T A L S

VEGETABLES   FRUIT   NUTS   WHOLE GRAINS

FUN	EMOTIONS	MOOD	ILLNESS	STRESS

Energy Level 1 2 3 4 5 6 7 8 9 10

MOVEMENT

Time of Day   Comments

Walking _____ steps/minutes

Weights _____ lbs, _____ reps

Stretches _____ minutes

Laughter _____

Other _____ **Weight** _____

BLOOD GLUCOSE NUMBERS

Time	Breakfast		Lunch		Dinner		Bedtime
	Before	After	Before	After	Before	After	

MEDICATIONS

Time	Type

Food for Those In Need

Better than food stamps are farmers' market coupons, making fresh fruits and vegetables available to those who cannot otherwise afford them. These coupons are distributed monthly through the Women, Infant, and Children Program. The program also supports farmers. In 40 states, 10,000 small farmers and 1 1/2 million women and children participate in this program—and eat 25% more fruits and vegetables!

Benefits of Farmers' Market Coupons/Programs

People using the coupons get to know the farmers and better understand where fruits and vegetables come from. Farmers are pleased with the success of the program for many reasons; income goes up 30–40% in some cases, and they love to see the children coming into the markets. The number of farmers' markets in the country has increased from 1,000 to 3,000, and there are many more in inner-city areas.

—**August Schumacher**
Undersecretary, Farm and Foreign Agricultural
Services, U.S. Government

Date _____ Deep Breathing _____ Sleep _____
                                                                    HOURS
Water ☐ ☐ ☐ ☐ ☐ ☐ ☐ ☐   Blood Pressure _____

F O O D

BREAKFAST   Time _____ Total Carb_____

      Serving Size   Food and Drinks

Grain
Vegetable
Protein
Fruit
Milk
Fat

SNACK   Time _____ Total Carb_____

LUNCH   Time _____ Total Carb_____

      Serving Size   Food and Drinks

Grain
Vegetable
Protein
Fruit
Milk
Fat

SNACK   Time _____ Total Carb_____

DINNER   Time _____ Total Carb_____

      Serving Size   Food and Drinks

Grain
Vegetable
Protein
Fruit
Milk
Fat

TOTALS

VEGETABLES   FRUIT   NUTS   WHOLE GRAINS

FUN	EMOTIONS	MOOD	ILLNESS	STRESS

Energy Level   1   2   3   4   5   6   7   8   9   10

MOVEMENT

Time of Day   Comments

Walking _____ steps/minutes

Weights _____ lbs, _____ reps

Stretches _____ minutes

Laughter _____

Other _____   **Weight** _____

BLOOD GLUCOSE NUMBERS

Time	Breakfast		Lunch		Dinner		Bedtime
	Before	After	Before	After	Before	After	

MEDICATIONS

Time	Type

Fare Start

"The major cause for a person being homeless usually starts when a person is young and does not have hope for a better alternative."

How can you make a difference in a person's life that is homeless?
You do not have to give them money to show respect or that you care. Smile.
Look for a way to be respectful, saying "Hello" or having a short conversation or giving them a smile is often the most appropriate action you can take.

—Cheryl Sesnon
Executive Director
The Fare Start Program, Seattle, WA

Date _____ Deep Breathing _____ Sleep _____
HOURS

Water 🥛 🥛 🥛 🥛 🥛 🥛 🥛 🥛 Blood Pressure _____

F O O D

BREAKFAST   Time _____ Total Carb_____

        Serving Size   Food and Drinks

Grain
Vegetable
Protein
Fruit
Milk
Fat

SNACK   Time _____ Total Carb_____

LUNCH   Time _____ Total Carb_____

        Serving Size   Food and Drinks

Grain
Vegetable
Protein
Fruit
Milk
Fat

SNACK   Time _____ Total Carb_____

DINNER   Time _____ Total Carb_____

        Serving Size   Food and Drinks

Grain
Vegetable
Protein
Fruit
Milk
Fat

T O T A L S

VEGETABLES   FRUIT   NUTS   WHOLE GRAINS

Energy Level   1   2   3   4   5   6   7   8   9   10

MOVEMENT

Time of Day   Comments

Walking _____ steps/minutes

Weights _____ lbs, _____ reps

Stretches _____ minutes

Laughter _____

Other _____   **Weight** _____

BLOOD GLUCOSE NUMBERS

Time	Breakfast		Lunch		Dinner		Bedtime
	Before	After	Before	After	Before	After	

MEDICATIONS

Time	Type

Celebrating the Family

Benefits of gathering the family at the table:

- Peace from being part of a family
- Comfort in conversation
- Knowledge of what children are doing
- Freedom of expression—you can ask about your children's day
- Opportunity to have one-on-one conversations
- Opening to discuss and help children resolve problems
- More nutritious meals because you serve fruits, vegetables, and home-made dishes

—David St. John Grubb and Cathy Powers

Date _____ Deep Breathing _____ Sleep _____
                                                                    HOURS

Water ☐ ☐ ☐ ☐ ☐ ☐ ☐ ☐   Blood Pressure _____

F O O D

BREAKFAST   Time _____ Total Carb_____

      Serving Size   Food and Drinks

Grain
Vegetable
Protein
Fruit
Milk
Fat

SNACK   Time _____ Total Carb_____

LUNCH   Time _____ Total Carb_____

      Serving Size   Food and Drinks

Grain
Vegetable
Protein
Fruit
Milk
Fat

SNACK   Time _____ Total Carb_____

DINNER   Time _____ Total Carb_____

      Serving Size   Food and Drinks

Grain
Vegetable
Protein
Fruit
Milk
Fat

T O T A L S

VEGETABLES   FRUIT   NUTS   WHOLE GRAINS

| FUN | EMOTIONS | MOOD | ILLNESS | STRESS |

Energy Level 1 2 3 4 5 6 7 8 9 10

MOVEMENT

Time of Day   Comments

Walking _____ steps/minutes

Weights _____ lbs, _____ reps

Stretches _____ minutes

Laughter _____

Other _____   **Weight** _____

BLOOD GLUCOSE NUMBERS

Time	Breakfast		Lunch		Dinner		Bedtime
	Before	After	Before	After	Before	After	

MEDICATIONS

Time	Type

Celebrating the Family

Ways to make the family meal a top priority:

- Let everyone participate in planning meals.
- Go to the grocery store together—it can be fun.
- Kids can help with meal planning and will participate more if they are involved.
- Let the children chop vegetables and set the table.
- Maintain a well-stocked pantry. If it is not there, you won't be able to cook it. Stock whole grains and other basic ingredients.
- Having foods partially prepared so the meal can be on the table in a short amount of time is a great help. A great example is having pizza dough and toppings prepared beforehand or using a slow-cooker to have the meal ready when you all get home.

—David St. John Grubb and Cathy Powers

Date _____ Deep Breathing _____ Sleep _____
HOURS

Water 🥛 🥛 🥛 🥛 🥛 🥛 🥛 🥛 Blood Pressure _____

F O O D

BREAKFAST　　　　　　Time _____ Total Carb_____

	Serving Size	Food and Drinks
Grain		
Vegetable		
Protein		
Fruit		
Milk		
Fat		

SNACK　　　　　　　　Time _____ Total Carb_____

LUNCH　　　　　　　　Time _____ Total Carb_____

	Serving Size	Food and Drinks
Grain		
Vegetable		
Protein		
Fruit		
Milk		
Fat		

SNACK　　　　　　　　Time _____ Total Carb_____

DINNER　　　　　　　Time _____ Total Carb_____

	Serving Size	Food and Drinks
Grain		
Vegetable		
Protein		
Fruit		
Milk		
Fat		

T O T A L S

VEGETABLES　　　FRUIT　　　NUTS　　　WHOLE GRAINS

FUN	EMOTIONS	MOOD	ILLNESS	STRESS

Energy Level 1 2 3 4 5 6 7 8 9 10

MOVEMENT

Time of Day   Comments

Walking _____ steps/minutes

Weights _____ lbs, _____ reps

Stretches _____ minutes

Laughter _____

Other _____   **Weight** _____

BLOOD GLUCOSE NUMBERS						
	Breakfast		Lunch		Dinner	
Time	Before	After	Before	After	Before	After	Bedtime

MEDICATIONS	
Time	Type

Cancer

We can prevent up to 35% of cancers with eating better and changing lifestyles, including more exercise. In the past years, there has been a downturn in cancer rates because of prevention, early detection, and good cancer treatments—but mostly it's due to prevention when people change lifestyle factors including diet and exercise. More than 100 substances in fruits and vegetables can help fight against cancer. These combinations are unique to fresh fruits and vegetables and probably cannot be mimicked by a vitamin supplement.

Are we eating enough fruits and veggies? No. In the U.S., only about half of the adults eat even four servings a day and the kids only three, which is a call to action to reach the goal of 5 or more a day for everyone! Eating fruits and vegetables is probably the easiest thing you can do for health, and your opportunities for prevention are enormous!

—**Gloria Stables, RD**
Director, Five A Day For Better Health,
National Cancer Institute

Date _____ Deep Breathing _____ Sleep _____
HOURS

Water ☐ ☐ ☐ ☐ ☐ ☐ ☐ ☐   Blood Pressure _____

F O O D

BREAKFAST   Time _____   Total Carb_____

	Serving Size	Food and Drinks
Grain		
Vegetable		
Protein		
Fruit		
Milk		
Fat		

SNACK   Time _____   Total Carb_____

LUNCH   Time _____   Total Carb_____

	Serving Size	Food and Drinks
Grain		
Vegetable		
Protein		
Fruit		
Milk		
Fat		

SNACK   Time _____   Total Carb_____

DINNER   Time _____   Total Carb_____

	Serving Size	Food and Drinks
Grain		
Vegetable		
Protein		
Fruit		
Milk		
Fat		

TOTALS

VEGETABLES   FRUIT   NUTS   WHOLE GRAINS

| FUN | EMOTIONS | MOOD | ILLNESS | STRESS |

Energy Level 1 2 3 4 5 6 7 8 9 10

MOVEMENT

Time of Day   Comments

Walking _____ steps/minutes

Weights _____ lbs, _____ reps

Stretches _____ minutes

Laughter _____

Other _____   **Weight** _____

BLOOD GLUCOSE NUMBERS

Time	Breakfast		Lunch		Dinner		Bedtime
	Before	After	Before	After	Before	After	

MEDICATIONS

Time	Type

Cancer

A serving of fruits and vegetables equals: 1 small fruit, 1/2 cup cut up fruit or cooked vegetable, 1 cup green leafy vegetable, 1/4 cup dried fruit, or 6 oz juice. Five servings of fruits and vegetables a day is a minimum goal, we now recommend nine servings a day!

- Buy fruits and vegetables and serve them, so they will be eaten.
- Have fruit servings at breakfast (fruit on your cereal).
- At every meal have at least one serving of a fruit or vegetable.
- Start your kids eating fruits and vegetables, so it becomes a routine for good health.

Find out which fruits and vegetables your family likes. There are over 270 varieties of fruits and vegetables. Try new ones and new ways to serve them, and enjoy the health that comes with these dynamic foods!

—Gloria Stables, RD
Director, Five A Day For Better Health,
National Cancer Institute
www.5aday.gov

Date _____ Deep Breathing _____ Sleep _____

HOURS

Water ☐ ☐ ☐ ☐ ☐ ☐ ☐ ☐ Blood Pressure _____

F O O D

BREAKFAST   Time _____ Total Carb_____

       Serving Size   Food and Drinks

Grain
Vegetable
Protein
Fruit
Milk
Fat

SNACK   Time _____ Total Carb_____

LUNCH   Time _____ Total Carb_____

       Serving Size   Food and Drinks

Grain
Vegetable
Protein
Fruit
Milk
Fat

SNACK   Time _____ Total Carb_____

DINNER   Time _____ Total Carb_____

       Serving Size   Food and Drinks

Grain
Vegetable
Protein
Fruit
Milk
Fat

TOTALS

VEGETABLES   FRUIT   NUTS   WHOLE GRAINS

| FUN | EMOTIONS | MOOD | ILLNESS | STRESS |

Energy Level 1 2 3 4 5 6 7 8 9 10

MOVEMENT

Time of Day   Comments

Walking _____ steps/minutes

Weights _____ lbs, _____ reps

Stretches _____ minutes

Laughter _____

Other _____   **Weight** _____

BLOOD GLUCOSE NUMBERS

Time	Breakfast		Lunch		Dinner		Bedtime
	Before	After	Before	After	Before	After	

MEDICATIONS

Time	Type

Tailored Cookbooks

Tailored Eating Plans

Family and personal food preferences can be used to create a tailored plan that can help individuals prepare foods healthfully and be more successful with their health behaviors.

People can more easily reduce fat in their diet with tailored information.

Recipes can be tailored to meet the whole family's needs.

Time constraints and skill level of the individual will be determined and figured into the tailored cookbook.

Can help people prevent disease before it starts.

Determine barriers to making behavior change so that these can be addressed as part of the eating plan.

—Vic Strecher, MD, MPH
Director, Health Media Research Labs,
University of Michigan

Date _____ Deep Breathing _____ Sleep _____
                                                                        HOURS
Water ⊓ ⊓ ⊓ ⊓ ⊓ ⊓ ⊓ ⊓   Blood Pressure _____

F O O D

BREAKFAST   Time _____ Total Carb_____

        Serving Size   Food and Drinks
Grain
Vegetable
Protein
Fruit
Milk
Fat

SNACK   Time _____ Total Carb_____

LUNCH   Time _____ Total Carb_____

        Serving Size   Food and Drinks
Grain
Vegetable
Protein
Fruit
Milk
Fat

SNACK   Time _____ Total Carb_____

DINNER   Time _____ Total Carb_____

        Serving Size   Food and Drinks
Grain
Vegetable
Protein
Fruit
Milk
Fat

T O T A L S

VEGETABLES   FRUIT   NUTS   WHOLE GRAINS

FUN	EMOTIONS	MOOD	ILLNESS	STRESS

Energy Level 1 2 3 4 5 6 7 8 9 10

MOVEMENT

Time of Day   Comments

Walking _____ steps/minutes

Weights _____ lbs, _____ reps

Stretches _____ minutes

Laughter _____

Other _____   **Weight** _____

BLOOD GLUCOSE NUMBERS

Time	Breakfast		Lunch		Dinner		Bedtime
	Before	After	Before	After	Before	After	

MEDICATIONS

Time	Type

Chocolate

As with all foods, chocolate can be a part of a healthy diet when you understand and practice moderation. Chocolate—as you probably already know—has various properties that make it a desirable and pleasurable food for those who "crave" it and those who just enjoy it. Chocolate will continue to be enjoyed as an ending to a meal, a token of love, or for a festive occasion— and someday, it may be enjoyed because of its relationship to health. Chocolate, especially dark chocolate, has monounsaturated fat—a good fat—and eating a bit of it makes us feel good, like endorphins that are released with exercise do.

Approximately 1 to 1 1/2 oz chocolate is one serving. You need to pay attention to the serving size to fit chocolate into a healthy diet. Too much chocolate may make it difficult to maintain an ideal weight.

—Douglas L. Taren, PhD
Associate Professor, University of Arizona
College of Medicine
www.chocolateinfo.com

Date _____ Deep Breathing _____ Sleep _____
                                                          HOURS

Water ⊔ ⊔ ⊔ ⊔ ⊔ ⊔ ⊔ ⊔   Blood Pressure _____

F O O D

BREAKFAST
Time _____ Total Carb _____

       Serving Size   Food and Drinks

Grain
Vegetable
Protein
Fruit
Milk
Fat

SNACK
Time _____ Total Carb _____

LUNCH
Time _____ Total Carb _____

       Serving Size   Food and Drinks

Grain
Vegetable
Protein
Fruit
Milk
Fat

SNACK
Time _____ Total Carb _____

DINNER
Time _____ Total Carb _____

       Serving Size   Food and Drinks

Grain
Vegetable
Protein
Fruit
Milk
Fat

TOTALS

VEGETABLES   FRUIT   NUTS   WHOLE GRAINS

FUN	EMOTIONS	MOOD	ILLNESS	STRESS

Energy Level 1 2 3 4 5 6 7 8 9 10

MOVEMENT

Time of Day   Comments

Walking _____ steps/minutes

Weights _____ lbs, _____ reps

Stretches _____ minutes

Laughter _____

Other _____   Weight _____

BLOOD GLUCOSE NUMBERS

Time	Breakfast		Lunch		Dinner		Bedtime
	Before	After	Before	After	Before	After	

MEDICATIONS

Time	Type

Functional Foods

Functional Foods are foods we eat everyday that have been modified or enhanced in some way to make them more healthful. Examples include: cereals fortified with B vitamins and other nutrients, orange juice with calcium added, and eggs with omega-3 fatty acids (the hens are fed flaxseed). If you are willing to eat whole grain cereals with ground flaxseed on top and to seek out all the food sources of calcium besides milk, such as broccoli and beans, you don't need fortified foods, but most people do need them. When you eat whole foods—not processed foods—you get taste, texture, color, and nutrients!

With fortified foods the government decides that a food needs to be fortified, such as grains with B vitamins. Functional foods come from a manufacturer's decision to enhance the food to market it for the health benefit.

—Cyndi Thomson, PhD, RD
the Arizona Prevention Center, University of Arizona

Date _____ Deep Breathing _____ Sleep _____
HOURS

Water ⬜ ⬜ ⬜ ⬜ ⬜ ⬜ ⬜ ⬜ Blood Pressure _____

F O O D

BREAKFAST   Time _____ Total Carb_____

            Serving Size   Food and Drinks
Grain
Vegetable
Protein
Fruit
Milk
Fat

SNACK   Time _____ Total Carb_____

LUNCH   Time _____ Total Carb_____

            Serving Size   Food and Drinks
Grain
Vegetable
Protein
Fruit
Milk
Fat

SNACK   Time _____ Total Carb_____

DINNER   Time _____ Total Carb_____

            Serving Size   Food and Drinks
Grain
Vegetable
Protein
Fruit
Milk
Fat

TOTALS

VEGETABLES   FRUIT   NUTS   WHOLE GRAINS

FUN	EMOTIONS	MOOD	ILLNESS	STRESS

Energy Level 1 2 3 4 5 6 7 8 9 10

MOVEMENT

Time of Day   Comments

Walking _____ steps/minutes

Weights _____ lbs, _____ reps

Stretches _____ minutes

Laughter _____

Other _____   Weight _____

BLOOD GLUCOSE NUMBERS

Time	Breakfast		Lunch		Dinner		Bedtime
	Before	After	Before	After	Before	After	

MEDICATIONS

Time	Type

Good Nutrition

The nutrients that you as an individual need from food you eat are determined by your age, gender, state of health, and level of activity. A registered dietitian can help you design a personal meal plan that fits you, and adjust it for any stage of your life. Whole foods and the nutrients we receive from these foods cannot be copied with pills, so focus on getting your best nutrition from food.

It's not so hard. Look for foods that have not been changed much by a manufacturer. At the supermarket, look for the colors of the rainbow in fruits and vegetables, which lead you to wise choices and lots of nutrition-dense foods.

—Cyndi Thomson, PhD, RD
University of Arizona

For more information: www.eatright.org

Date _____ Deep Breathing _____ Sleep _____
                                                                              HOURS
Water ☐ ☐ ☐ ☐ ☐ ☐ ☐ ☐   Blood Pressure _____

F O O D

BREAKFAST   Time _____ Total Carb_____

     Serving Size   Food and Drinks
Grain
Vegetable
Protein
Fruit
Milk
Fat

SNACK   Time _____ Total Carb_____

LUNCH   Time _____ Total Carb_____

     Serving Size   Food and Drinks
Grain
Vegetable
Protein
Fruit
Milk
Fat

SNACK   Time _____ Total Carb_____

DINNER   Time _____ Total Carb_____

     Serving Size   Food and Drinks
Grain
Vegetable
Protein
Fruit
Milk
Fat

T O T A L S

VEGETABLES   FRUIT   NUTS   WHOLE GRAINS

Energy Level   1   2   3   4   5   6   7   8   9   10

MOVEMENT

Time of Day   Comments

Walking _____ steps/minutes

Weights _____ lbs, _____ reps

Stretches _____ minutes

Laughter _____

Other _____   Weight _____

	BLOOD GLUCOSE NUMBERS								MEDICATIONS	
	Breakfast		Lunch		Dinner				Time	Type
Time	Before	After	Before	After	Before	After	Bedtime			

Folate

Folate is an essential B vitamin involved in every single cell in our body. It is important for preventing heart disease. It is important for women of child-bearing age, because 400 mcg of folate a day protects unborn babies from neural birth defects such as cleft palate and spina bifida. In fact, over 50% of these birth defects could be prevented with folate.

In the U.S., foods with flour must be enriched with folic acid, the man-made version of folate. The recommendation is for adults to eat 400 mcg folate daily. Do you?

Foods high in folate:

Beans are the best source   Most dark leafy greens
Broccoli   Orange juice
Strawberries   Frozen boysenberries
Asparagus

—Evelyn Tribole, MS, RD
Author, *Stealth Health*

Date _____ Deep Breathing _____ Sleep _____
HOURS

Water ▯ ▯ ▯ ▯ ▯ ▯ ▯ ▯   Blood Pressure _____

F O O D

BREAKFAST   Time _____ Total Carb_____

Serving Size	Food and Drinks
Grain	
Vegetable	
Protein	
Fruit	
Milk	
Fat	

SNACK   Time _____ Total Carb_____

LUNCH   Time _____ Total Carb_____

Serving Size	Food and Drinks
Grain	
Vegetable	
Protein	
Fruit	
Milk	
Fat	

SNACK   Time _____ Total Carb_____

DINNER   Time _____ Total Carb_____

Serving Size	Food and Drinks
Grain	
Vegetable	
Protein	
Fruit	
Milk	
Fat	

TOTALS

VEGETABLES   FRUIT   NUTS   WHOLE GRAINS

FUN	EMOTIONS	MOOD	ILLNESS	STRESS

Energy Level 1 2 3 4 5 6 7 8 9 10

MOVEMENT

Time of Day   Comments

Walking _____ steps/minutes

Weights _____ lbs, _____ reps

Stretches _____ minutes

Laughter _____

Other _____   **Weight** _____

BLOOD GLUCOSE NUMBERS

Time	Breakfast		Lunch		Dinner		Bedtime
	Before	After	Before	After	Before	After	

MEDICATIONS

Time	Type

Carb Counting

All carbohydrates (sugars and starches) are equal in the way your body views them. When carbohydrates (carbs) enter the bloodstream, they have all been broken down into glucose, and insulin allows the glucose to get into the body's cells to be used for energy.

Refined carbs, such as sugar and white flour, raise your blood glucose and contribute energy but don't have many vitamins and minerals, which you need. To eat less of these:

- Look at the ingredient list to see where the sweetness is coming from
- Avoid empty calories from high fructose corn syrup and sweetened beverages
- Eat fruit instead of drinking juice
- Drink more water—no sugar and no calories
- Choose a beverage that has some nutrition (100% juice gives you some vitamins)
- Try a diet version (may be artificially sweetened) but water and tea are better choices

—Hope S. Warshaw, MMSc, RD, CDE
Author, *Diabetes Meal Planning Made Easy* and
The ADA Guide to Healthy Restaurant Eating

Date _____ Deep Breathing _____ Sleep _____

HOURS

Water 🥛 🥛 🥛 🥛 🥛 🥛 🥛 🥛 Blood Pressure _____

F O O D

BREAKFAST Time _____ Total Carb_____

Serving Size	Food and Drinks
Grain	
Vegetable	
Protein	
Fruit	
Milk	
Fat	

SNACK Time _____ Total Carb_____

LUNCH Time _____ Total Carb_____

Serving Size	Food and Drinks
Grain	
Vegetable	
Protein	
Fruit	
Milk	
Fat	

SNACK Time _____ Total Carb_____

DINNER Time _____ Total Carb_____

Serving Size	Food and Drinks
Grain	
Vegetable	
Protein	
Fruit	
Milk	
Fat	

T O T A L S

VEGETABLES   FRUIT   NUTS   WHOLE GRAINS

FUN	EMOTIONS	MOOD	ILLNESS	STRESS

Energy Level 1 2 3 4 5 6 7 8 9 10

MOVEMENT

Time of Day   Comments

Walking _____ steps/minutes

Weights _____ lbs, _____ reps

Stretches _____ minutes

Laughter _____

Other _____   **Weight** _____

BLOOD GLUCOSE NUMBERS

Time	Breakfast		Lunch		Dinner		Bedtime
	Before	After	Before	After	Before	After	

MEDICATIONS

Time	Type

Fructose and Honey

Do **fructose** and **honey** have fewer calories than sugar? No, they are the same. Fructose causes a slightly lower rise in blood glucose, but calorie for calorie, it is the same as sugar. When you are hungry for something sweet:

- Set goals, such as have a sweet one or two times a week.
- Fresh fruit and dried fruit are healthier choices that may satisfy the sweet tooth.
- Split desserts with others to keep calories in check.

Altering recipes to reduce the sugar:
Use recipes as a guideline, since they are often ripe for improving! Usually you can leave out 1/3–1/2 of the sugar or sweetener. Try this; the result is often just as delicious but cuts down the risk!

—**Hope S. Warshaw, MMSc, RD, CDE**
Author, *Diabetes Meal Planning Made Easy* and
The ADA Guide to Healthy Restaurant Eating

Date _____ Deep Breathing _____ Sleep _____
HOURS

Water ☐ ☐ ☐ ☐ ☐ ☐ ☐ ☐   Blood Pressure _____

F O O D

BREAKFAST   Time _____ Total Carb_____

	Serving Size	Food and Drinks
Grain		
Vegetable		
Protein		
Fruit		
Milk		
Fat		

SNACK   Time _____ Total Carb_____

LUNCH   Time _____ Total Carb_____

	Serving Size	Food and Drinks
Grain		
Vegetable		
Protein		
Fruit		
Milk		
Fat		

SNACK   Time _____ Total Carb_____

DINNER   Time _____ Total Carb_____

	Serving Size	Food and Drinks
Grain		
Vegetable		
Protein		
Fruit		
Milk		
Fat		

TOTALS

VEGETABLES   FRUIT   NUTS   WHOLE GRAINS

Energy Level 1 2 3 4 5 6 7 8 9 10

MOVEMENT

Time of Day   Comments

Walking _____ steps/minutes

Weights _____ lbs, _____ reps

Stretches _____ minutes

Laughter _____

Other _____   **Weight** _____

BLOOD GLUCOSE NUMBERS

Time	Breakfast		Lunch		Dinner		Bedtime
	Before	After	Before	After	Before	After	

MEDICATIONS

Time	Type

Using Artificial Sweeteners

Artificial sweeteners have been researched extensively to be sure they are safe for consumers. When you use sweeteners, make sure the government has tested and approves them. As with all foods, these sweeteners can fit into a balanced and varied diet and should be consumed in moderation. Too much artificial sweetener can cause stomach upsets and gastric distress—as some people have learned to their dismay.

You might want to experiment with natural low-calorie sweeteners, such as stevia, which is a plant whose leaves are 300 times sweeter than sugar, but no aftertaste, no calories, and no rise in blood glucose. One leaf in a pitcher of tea makes it quite sweet.

—Hope S. Warshaw, MMSc, RD, CDE
Author, *Diabetes Meal Planning Made Easy* and
The ADA Guide to Healthy Restaurant Eating

Date _____ Deep Breathing _____ Sleep _____
_{HOURS}

Water ⬜ ⬜ ⬜ ⬜ ⬜ ⬜ ⬜ ⬜   Blood Pressure _____

F O O D

BREAKFAST   Time _____ Total Carb_____

Serving Size   Food and Drinks

Grain
Vegetable
Protein
Fruit
Milk
Fat

SNACK   Time _____ Total Carb_____

LUNCH   Time _____ Total Carb_____

Serving Size   Food and Drinks

Grain
Vegetable
Protein
Fruit
Milk
Fat

SNACK   Time _____ Total Carb_____

DINNER   Time _____ Total Carb_____

Serving Size   Food and Drinks

Grain
Vegetable
Protein
Fruit
Milk
Fat

T O T A L S

VEGETABLES   FRUIT   NUTS   WHOLE GRAINS

FUN	EMOTIONS	MOOD	ILLNESS	STRESS

Energy Level 1 2 3 4 5 6 7 8 9 10

MOVEMENT

Time of Day   Comments

Walking _____ steps/minutes

Weights _____ lbs, _____ reps

Stretches _____ minutes

Laughter _____

Other _____

Weight _____

BLOOD GLUCOSE NUMBERS

Time	Breakfast		Lunch		Dinner		Bedtime
	Before	After	Before	After	Before	After	

MEDICATIONS

Time	Type

Calcium

Calcium is critical. One in 4 women will get osteoporosis (porous bones). Blood calcium levels must be maintained at all times, so if you don't get calcium in the diet, your body will draw the calcium from your bones, which can lead to osteoporosis. There are two key elements to develop and maintain your bones: weight-bearing exercise and eating foods with calcium. You deposit about half of your adult bone skeleton in a few adolescent years, so exercising and consuming adequate calcium makes all the difference.

Adults need 1,000 mg a day but most get about 500 mg a day.
Adolescents need between 1,200 and 1,500 mg daily.
Women over 50 need 1,200 mg a day, but most average 400 mg a day.

The best way to get calcium is through food because these foods also contain important nutrients including magnesium, vitamin D, riboflavin, vitamin A, phosphorous, and protein.

—Connie Weaver, PhD
Department Head, Food and Nutrition, Purdue University

Date _____ Deep Breathing _____ Sleep _____
HOURS

Water ▭ ▭ ▭ ▭ ▭ ▭ ▭ ▭   Blood Pressure _____

F O O D

BREAKFAST   Time _____ Total Carb_____

Serving Size   Food and Drinks

Grain
Vegetable
Protein
Fruit
Milk
Fat

SNACK   Time _____ Total Carb_____

LUNCH   Time _____ Total Carb_____

Serving Size   Food and Drinks

Grain
Vegetable
Protein
Fruit
Milk
Fat

SNACK   Time _____ Total Carb_____

DINNER   Time _____ Total Carb_____

Serving Size   Food and Drinks

Grain
Vegetable
Protein
Fruit
Milk
Fat

TOTALS

VEGETABLES   FRUIT   NUTS   WHOLE GRAINS

FUN	EMOTIONS	MOOD	ILLNESS	STRESS

Energy Level 1 2 3 4 5 6 7 8 9 10

MOVEMENT

Time of Day   Comments

Walking _____ steps/minutes

Weights _____ lbs, _____ reps

Stretches _____ minutes

Laughter _____

Other _____   **Weight** _____

BLOCK GLUCOSE NUMBERS								MEDICATIONS	
	Breakfast		Lunch		Dinner			Time	Type
Time	Before	After	Before	After	Before	After	Bedtime		

Dairy Foods

Dairy foods are an important source of calcium. A serving of low-fat milk, yogurt, or cheese with every meal is recommended. Research shows calcium can help prevent a person from gaining weight. You can use fortified foods, such as calcium fortified orange juice. It is difficult to get enough calcium in foods such as greens and broccoli (you would need 4 1/2 servings to match one glass of milk), but it can be done.

If you cannot get calcium through foods or you are lactose intolerant, you can take supplements. Calcium from most supplements is absorbed as well as from milk. Viactiv is a soft chewable that is a great calcium source, especially for people who do not like to swallow large tablets (1 Viactiv chew contains 500 mg per serving). Some research indicates that calcium is better absorbed when taken with magnesium in a 2 to 1 ratio (500 mg calcium to 250 mg magnesium). The upper limit of calcium is 2,500 mg day; this would be difficult to achieve with food.

—Connie Weaver, PhD
Head, Food and Nutrition, Purdue University

Date _____ Deep Breathing _____ Sleep _____
HOURS

Water ⬜ ⬜ ⬜ ⬜ ⬜ ⬜ ⬜ ⬜   Blood Pressure _____

F O O D

BREAKFAST   Time _____ Total Carb_____

Serving Size	Food and Drinks
Grain	
Vegetable	
Protein	
Fruit	
Milk	
Fat	

SNACK   Time _____ Total Carb_____

LUNCH   Time _____ Total Carb_____

Serving Size	Food and Drinks
Grain	
Vegetable	
Protein	
Fruit	
Milk	
Fat	

SNACK   Time _____ Total Carb_____

DINNER   Time _____ Total Carb_____

Serving Size	Food and Drinks
Grain	
Vegetable	
Protein	
Fruit	
Milk	
Fat	

T O T A L S

VEGETABLES   FRUIT   NUTS   WHOLE GRAINS

Energy Level   1   2   3   4   5   6   7   8   9   10

MOVEMENT

Time of Day   Comments

Walking _____ steps/minutes

Weights _____ lbs, _____ reps

Stretches _____ minutes

Laughter _____

Other _____   **Weight** _____

BLOOD GLUCOSE NUMBERS

Time	Breakfast		Lunch		Dinner		Bedtime
	Before	After	Before	After	Before	After	

MEDICATIONS

Time	Type

Chinese Cooking

Chinese cooking is simple, fresh, and healthy. It focuses on rice, noodles, and vegetables, with meat used as a flavoring. It is quite low in fat and takes little time to prepare.

The basic flavor profile is simple yet profound, and you can create almost anything with these flavorings:

ginger	oyster sauce
garlic	hoisin
green onion	rice vinegar
soy sauce	five spice powder
sesame oil	

The most important kitchen tool is a knife, particularly for Asian cuisine.

—**Martin Yan**
Host: *Yan Can Cook* TV show
Culinary Ambassador of East Asia cooking to the Western World

Date _____ Deep Breathing _____ Sleep _____
HOURS

Water ⬚ ⬚ ⬚ ⬚ ⬚ ⬚ ⬚ ⬚   Blood Pressure _____

F O O D

BREAKFAST　　　　　Time _____ Total Carb_____

　　　　　Serving Size　　Food and Drinks

Grain
Vegetable
Protein
Fruit
Milk
Fat

SNACK　　　　　　　Time _____ Total Carb_____

LUNCH　　　　　　　Time _____ Total Carb_____

　　　　　Serving Size　　Food and Drinks

Grain
Vegetable
Protein
Fruit
Milk
Fat

SNACK　　　　　　　Time _____ Total Carb_____

DINNER　　　　　　Time _____ Total Carb_____

　　　　　Serving Size　　Food and Drinks

Grain
Vegetable
Protein
Fruit
Milk
Fat

TOTALS

VEGETABLES　　　　　FRUIT　　　　NUTS　　　WHOLE GRAINS

FUN	EMOTIONS	MOOD	ILLNESS	STRESS

Energy Level   1   2   3   4   5   6   7   8   9   10

MOVEMENT

Time of Day   Comments

Walking _____ steps/minutes

Weights _____ lbs, _____ reps

Stretches _____ minutes

Laughter _____

Other _____   **Weight** _____

BLOOD GLUCOSE NUMBERS

Time	Breakfast		Lunch		Dinner		Bedtime
	Before	After	Before	After	Before	After	

MEDICATIONS

Time	Type

Health and Food Trends of the Chinese People

- Very few Chinese are overweight.
- Typical menu has noodles in the north and rice in the south and a lot of vegetables for both areas. Food is mostly vegetarian, and meat and shellfish are used as flavoring.
- The Chinese are more stressed these days, and the diet is changing, but overall there is less sugar, cream, and butter in their diet than compared to the common diet in the United States. Fresh fruit is dessert, and it is very likely that the people are healthy as a result.
- The Chinese people walk, ride bikes, and do traditional exercises like Tai Chi all their lives long.

—Martin Yan
Host: *Yan Can Cook*, Food and Restaurant
Consultant and Culinary Ambassador of East Asia
cooking to the Western World

For more information: www.yancancook.com

Date _____ Deep Breathing _____ Sleep _____

HOURS

Water ▯ ▯ ▯ ▯ ▯ ▯ ▯ ▯   Blood Pressure _____

F O O D

BREAKFAST   Time _____ Total Carb_____

	Serving Size	Food and Drinks
Grain		
Vegetable		
Protein		
Fruit		
Milk		
Fat		

SNACK   Time _____ Total Carb_____

LUNCH   Time _____ Total Carb_____

	Serving Size	Food and Drinks
Grain		
Vegetable		
Protein		
Fruit		
Milk		
Fat		

SNACK   Time _____ Total Carb_____

DINNER   Time _____ Total Carb_____

	Serving Size	Food and Drinks
Grain		
Vegetable		
Protein		
Fruit		
Milk		
Fat		

T O T A L S

VEGETABLES   FRUIT   NUTS   WHOLE GRAINS

| FUN | EMOTIONS | MOOD | ILLNESS | STRESS |

Energy Level   1   2   3   4   5   6   7   8   9   10

MOVEMENT

Time of Day   Comments

Walking _____ steps/minutes

Weights _____ lbs, _____ reps

Stretches _____ minutes

Laughter _____

Other _____

Weight _____

BLOOD GLUCOSE NUMBERS

Time	Breakfast		Lunch		Dinner		Bedtime
	Before	After	Before	After	Before	After	

MEDICATIONS

Time	Type

The Sizes of Servings

People underestimate how much food they eat. Food records are often underreported by 50% because people don't understand what a serving size is for each food. Portion sizes do vary within food categories. Breads are most confusing:

1 serving (1 oz) = 1 slice of bread, 1/2 cup of pasta, or 1 pretzel

The sizes of the foods are different depending on where you dine. For example,

- Many large bagels can be up to 5 bread servings.
- A ballgame pretzel is 5 bread servings.
- Most store-bought muffins are 5 or 6 bread servings, not to mention the fat content!
- One pasta dish in a restaurant can be 1,000 calories or more.

—Lisa R. Young, MS, RD, PhD

Date _____ Deep Breathing _____ Sleep _____

Water ☐ ☐ ☐ ☐ ☐ ☐ ☐ ☐   Blood Pressure _____   HOURS

F O O D

BREAKFAST   Time _____ Total Carb_____

	Serving Size	Food and Drinks
Grain		
Vegetable		
Protein		
Fruit		
Milk		
Fat		

SNACK   Time _____ Total Carb_____

LUNCH   Time _____ Total Carb_____

	Serving Size	Food and Drinks
Grain		
Vegetable		
Protein		
Fruit		
Milk		
Fat		

SNACK   Time _____ Total Carb_____

DINNER   Time _____ Total Carb_____

	Serving Size	Food and Drinks
Grain		
Vegetable		
Protein		
Fruit		
Milk		
Fat		

TOTALS

VEGETABLES   FRUIT   NUTS   WHOLE GRAINS

FUN	EMOTIONS	MOOD	ILLNESS	STRESS

Energy Level   1   2   3   4   5   6   7   8   9   10

MOVEMENT

Time of Day   Comments

Walking _____ steps/minutes

Weights _____ lbs, _____ reps

Stretches _____ minutes

Laughter _____

Other _____   Weight _____

BLOOD GLUCOSE NUMBERS								MEDICATIONS	
	Breakfast		Lunch		Dinner			Time	Type
Time	Before	After	Before	After	Before	After	Bedtime		

Portion Sizes

- Make it your responsibility to understand portion sizes.
- Learn easy ways to remember portion sizes, such as 3 oz meat = a deck of cards, a light bulb = a serving of vegetables, a slice of cheese = a domino.
- Plan ahead for meals; a steak is okay if you focus on eating grains, vegetables, and fruits the rest of the day.
- Buy smaller single-serving bags of chips or snacks; when people buy larger portions they eat the whole thing.
- When eating out, order appetizer portions, a salad, and a soup, or take half of your meal home.
- Tell the waiter you would like to split a meal or have a smaller portion, and then add more vegetables, salads, or side dishes.
- See a registered dietitian to learn more about portion sizes and techniques.

—Lisa R. Young, MS, RD, PhD

Date _____ Deep Breathing _____ Sleep _____

Water ☐ ☐ ☐ ☐ ☐ ☐ ☐ ☐   Blood Pressure _____

F O O D

BREAKFAST　　　　　Time _____ Total Carb_____

	Serving Size	Food and Drinks
Grain		
Vegetable		
Protein		
Fruit		
Milk		
Fat		

SNACK　　　　　　　Time _____ Total Carb_____

LUNCH　　　　　　　Time _____ Total Carb_____

	Serving Size	Food and Drinks
Grain		
Vegetable		
Protein		
Fruit		
Milk		
Fat		

SNACK　　　　　　　Time _____ Total Carb_____

DINNER　　　　　　　Time _____ Total Carb_____

	Serving Size	Food and Drinks
Grain		
Vegetable		
Protein		
Fruit		
Milk		
Fat		

T O T A L S

VEGETABLES　　　　　FRUIT　　　　NUTS　　　WHOLE GRAINS

FUN	EMOTIONS	MOOD	ILLNESS	STRESS

Energy Level   1   2   3   4   5   6   7   8   9   10

MOVEMENT

Time of Day   Comments

Walking _____ steps/minutes

Weights _____ lbs, _____ reps

Stretches _____ minutes

Laughter _____

Other _____   **Weight** _____

BLOOD GLUCOSE NUMBERS

Time	Breakfast		Lunch		Dinner		Bedtime
	Before	After	Before	After	Before	After	

MEDICATIONS

Time	Type

Truly Great Snacks

Snacking can nourish you—or be a source of calories and fat. Wise snacks, with an eye on portion size can provide great nutrition for children, teenagers, adults, and elders.

What makes a healthy snack?
- Calories and portion size should be reasonable.
- Snacks should include more than one food group—mostly good carbohydrates with a small amount of protein and fat.
- Fiber, as in fruit, vegetables, whole grains, and beans, and a bit of good fat, such as nuts, seeds, or olive oil, help you feel full and satisfied.
- Sweet drinks like sodas (and fruit juice) have too much sugar and leave you hungry.
- Snacks do not have to be traditional foods like pretzels, fruit, and popcorn; they can be leftovers, fruit smoothies, and cereals.
- Time your snacks so that you don't go more than five hours without eating.

—Kathleen Zelman, MPH, RD

Date _____ Deep Breathing _____ Sleep _____
HOURS

Water ☐ ☐ ☐ ☐ ☐ ☐ ☐ ☐   Blood Pressure _____

F O O D

BREAKFAST   Time _____ Total Carb_____

	Serving Size	Food and Drinks
Grain		
Vegetable		
Protein		
Fruit		
Milk		
Fat		

SNACK   Time _____ Total Carb_____

LUNCH   Time _____ Total Carb_____

	Serving Size	Food and Drinks
Grain		
Vegetable		
Protein		
Fruit		
Milk		
Fat		

SNACK   Time _____ Total Carb_____

DINNER   Time _____ Total Carb_____

	Serving Size	Food and Drinks
Grain		
Vegetable		
Protein		
Fruit		
Milk		
Fat		

TOTALS

VEGETABLES   FRUIT   NUTS   WHOLE GRAINS

| FUN | EMOTIONS | MOOD | ILLNESS | STRESS |

Energy Level 1 2 3 4 5 6 7 8 9 10

MOVEMENT

Time of Day   Comments

Walking _____ steps/minutes

Weights _____ lbs, _____ reps

Stretches _____ minutes

Laughter _____

Other _____   **Weight** _____

BLOOD GLUCOSE NUMBERS

Time	Breakfast		Lunch		Dinner		Bedtime
	Before	After	Before	After	Before	After	

MEDICATIONS

Time	Type

Munching Too Much?

Large, jumbo, and super-size portions have lots of calories and fat, like a super-size muffin at 400 calories and 30 grams of fat! Now there's a good reason to make your own! Opt for half an English muffin, fresh fruit, tea, or half of a higher-calorie choice.

Curb mindless munching:
Often we snack out of habit or without our wits about us. Maintain a level of consciousness so you know what you are eating. Never eat "out of the bag," since you don't know how much you are eating. Select the portion (Nutrition Facts label) and put the bag away.

Snacks to take with you:
Grains: cereal, crackers, and rice cakes in a single-serve container
Vegetables and fruit: fresh cut vegetables and fruit in zipper-lock storage bags
Milk/yogurt/cheese: cheese sticks, single-serve yogurts, milk boxes or smoothies in a thermos

—Kathleen Zelman, MPH, RD
American Dietetic Association Spokesperson

Emotions

ow you've spent 3 or 4 months with us trying some lifestyle changes. Fill this out for how you're feeling now. Then you can go back and compare it to how you felt when you began. It's such fun to see progress! Simply check the number after the feelings that best describe how you feel *TODAY*.

I'M GRATEFUL FOR THESE										
Loving	1	2	3	4	5	6	7	8	9	10
Joyful	1	2	3	4	5	6	7	8	9	10
Peaceful	1	2	3	4	5	6	7	8	9	10
Patient	1	2	3	4	5	6	7	8	9	10
Gentle	1	2	3	4	5	6	7	8	9	10
Ethical	1	2	3	4	5	6	7	8	9	10
Faithful	1	2	3	4	5	6	7	8	9	10
Mild Mannered	1	2	3	4	5	6	7	8	9	10
Self Controlled	1	2	3	4	5	6	7	8	9	10

I'M WORKING ON THESE										
Resentment	1	2	3	4	5	6	7	8	9	10
Despondent	1	2	3	4	5	6	7	8	9	10
Argumentative	1	2	3	4	5	6	7	8	9	10
Impatient	1	2	3	4	5	6	7	8	9	10
Impetuous	1	2	3	4	5	6	7	8	9	10
Abusive (Hurtful)	1	2	3	4	5	6	7	8	9	10
Unreliable	1	2	3	4	5	6	7	8	9	10
Conceited (Vain)	1	2	3	4	5	6	7	8	9	10
Dissatisfied	1	2	3	4	5	6	7	8	9	10

(1 = Less; 10 = More Obvious)

How to Use the Monthly Charts

rite the name of the month at the top. The first section is for weight changes over the month. You might weigh every morning, as Treena and I do, or only once a week. The centerline on the graph is your goal weight for that week, so you have to write that number on the left side. Then tick off five pounds above and below that line, one pound for each line. Measure across from the weight and down from the day you weighed and make a dot at the point those lines intersect. When you have put dots for each day you weighed, then you can get out your ruler and draw a line connecting the dots. If you see a wide or surprising swing, you can go back to your daily record and see what else was happening then. Were you on a business trip and eating out every meal? The trend of eating higher amounts of calories will show pretty quickly.

The next section is for recording blood sugar levels. Put a large dot for fasting glucose and a + sign for postprandial (2 hours after the first bite of the meal) checks. Again, move from the reading on the left and the day at the top and make the dot where those two lines meet. If you have wide swings, go back to your daily records and see whether you were ill, or traveling, or under a great deal of stress, or you started an enthusiastic exercise program that dropped your blood sugar to normal! You can note possible causes in the margin to discuss with your health care team when you meet.

The bottom two sections are for recording changes in blood pressure. The top section is for the top number (systolic) on your blood pressure, when your heart beats. The bottom section is for the bottom number (diastolic) on your blood pressure, when your heart is at rest. Again, you should see a connection between how well you are eating, sleeping, breathing, and exercising and your blood pressure levels.

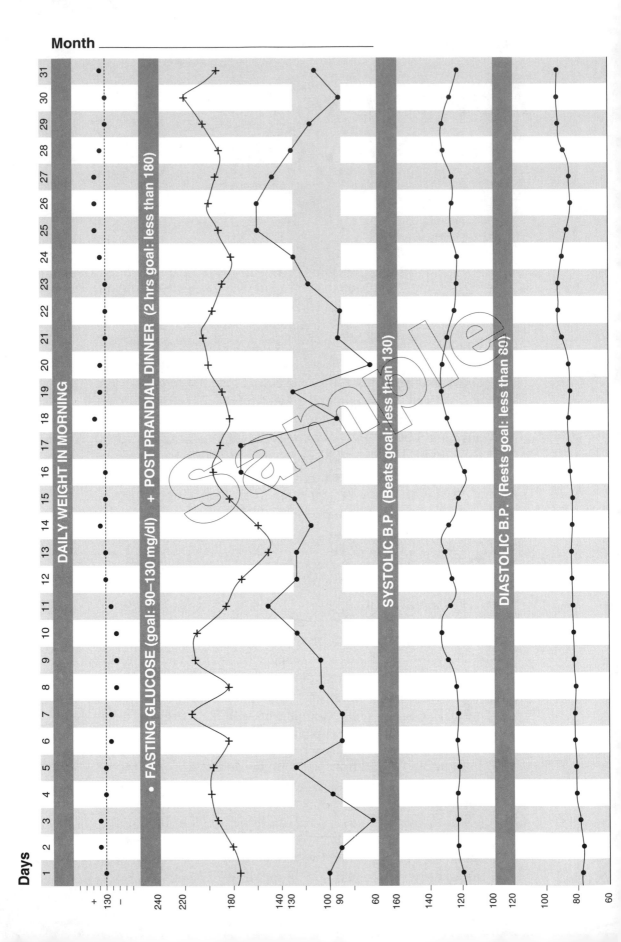

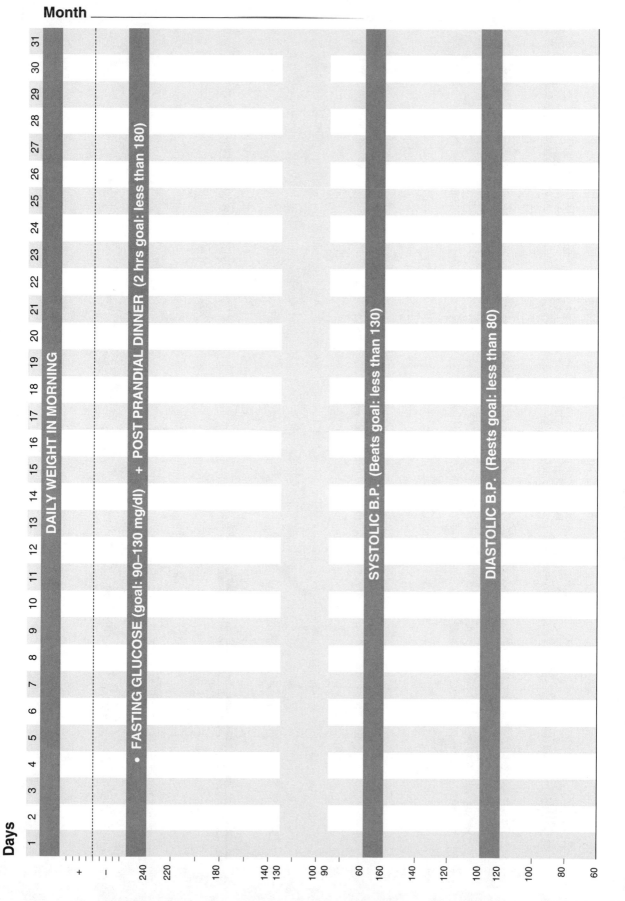

Month _____

Days

DAILY WEIGHT IN MORNING

• FASTING GLUCOSE (goal: 90–130 mg/dl) + POST PRANDIAL DINNER (2 hrs goal: less than 180)

SYSTOLIC B.P. (Beats goal: less than 130)

DIASTOLIC B.P. (Rests goal: less than 80)

Month _____

Days

	1	2	3	4	5	6	7	8	9	10	11	12	13	14	15	16	17	18	19	20	21	22	23	24	25	26	27	28	29	30	31

DAILY WEIGHT IN MORNING

+

−

• FASTING GLUCOSE (goal: 90–130 mg/dl) + POST PRANDIAL DINNER (2 hrs goal: less than 180)

240
220
180
140
130
100
90
60

SYSTOLIC B.P. (Beats goal: less than 130)

160
140
120
100

DIASTOLIC B.P. (Rests goal: less than 80)

120
100
80
60

Month _____

Days

| | 1 | 2 | 3 | 4 | 5 | 6 | 7 | 8 | 9 | 10 | 11 | 12 | 13 | 14 | 15 | 16 | 17 | 18 | 19 | 20 | 21 | 22 | 23 | 24 | 25 | 26 | 27 | 28 | 29 | 30 | 31 |

DAILY WEIGHT IN MORNING

+
–

• **FASTING GLUCOSE** (goal: 90–130 mg/dl)   + **POST PRANDIAL DINNER** (2 hrs goal: less than 180)

240
220
180
140
130
100
90
60

SYSTOLIC B.P. (Beats goal: less than 130)

160
140
120
100

DIASTOLIC B.P. (Rests goal: less than 80)

120
100
80
60

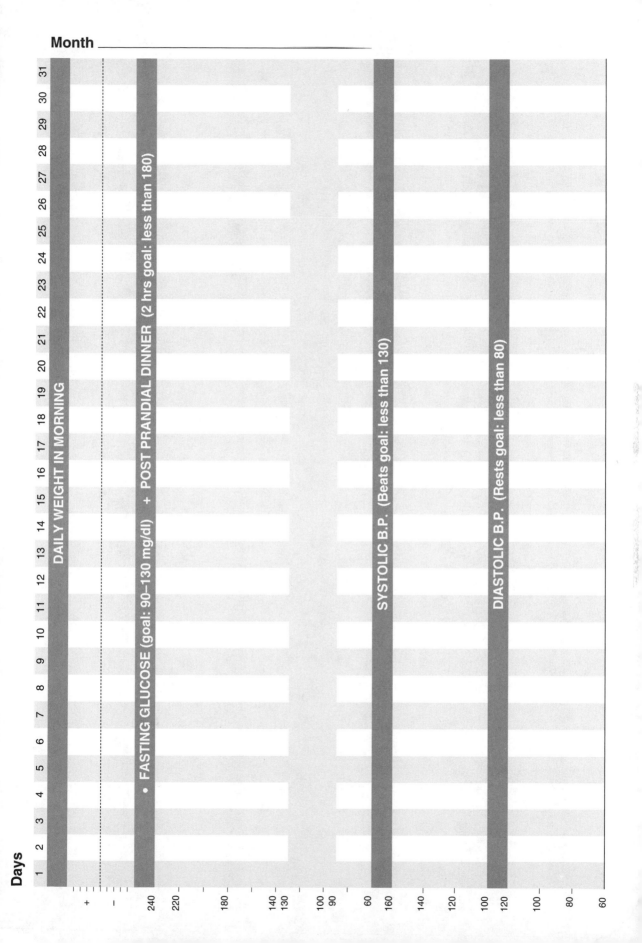

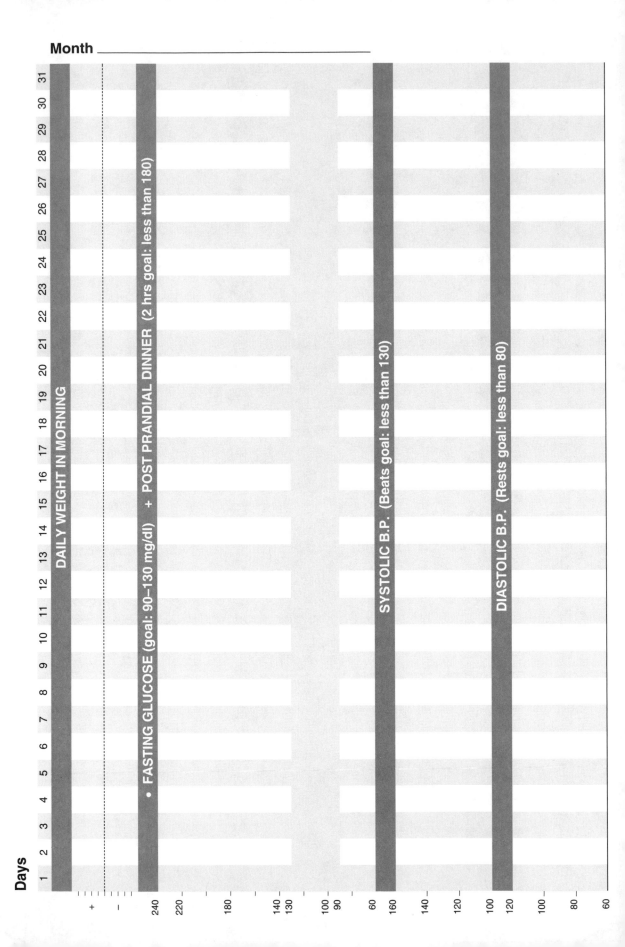

DATE: _____

My weight today is _____.

My blood pressure is _____.

My LDL (bad) cholesterol is _____.

My HDL (good) cholesterol is _____.

My triglyceride level is _____.

My AIC is _____.

My BG level is _____.

You can use the charts on the following pages to think about meal changes and exercise choices. Remember you have to think about change before you can do it. Have fun.

PERSONAL MENU SELECTIONS

MENU	CREATIVE ALTERNATIVES	POTENTIAL BENEFITS
BREAKFASTS		
LUNCHES		
SNACKS		

PERSONAL MENU SELECTIONS

MENU	CREATIVE ALTERNATIVES	POTENTIAL BENEFITS

DINNER

PERSONAL ACTIVITY SELECTIONS

ACTIVITY	DAILY	WEEKLY (# OF DAYS)	ONCE A WEEK	OCCASIONAL SUMMER	OCCASIONAL WINTER	ESTIMATED DAY SITTING	DO MORE!

About the American Diabetes Association

The American Diabetes Association is the nation's leading voluntary health organization supporting diabetes research, information, and advocacy. Its mission is to prevent and cure diabetes and to improve the lives of all people affected by diabetes. The American Diabetes Association is the leading publisher of comprehensive diabetes information. Its huge library of practical and authoritative books for people with diabetes covers every aspect of self-care—cooking and nutrition, fitness, weight control, medications, complications, emotional issues, and general self-care.

To order American Diabetes Association books: Call 1-800-232-6733. Or log on to http://store.diabetes.org

To join the American Diabetes Association: Call 1-800-806-7801. www.diabetes.org/membership

For more information about diabetes or ADA programs and services: Call 1-800-342-2383. E-mail: AskADA@diabetes.org or log on to www.diabetes.org

To locate an ADA/NCQA Recognized Provider of quality diabetes care in your area: www.ncqa.org/dprp/

To find an ADA Recognized Education Program in your area: Call 1-888-232-0822. www.diabetes.org/recognition/education.asp

To join the fight to increase funding for diabetes research, end discrimination, and improve insurance coverage: Call 1-800-342-2383. www.diabetes.org/advocacy

To find out how you can get involved with the programs in your community: Call 1-800-342-2383. See below for program Web addresses.

- *American Diabetes Month:* Educational activities aimed at those diagnosed with diabetes—month of November. www.diabetes.org/ADM
- *American Diabetes Alert:* Annual public awareness campaign to find the undiagnosed—held the fourth Tuesday in March. www.diabetes.org/alert
- *The Diabetes Assistance & Resources Program (DAR):* diabetes awareness program targeted to the Latino community. www.diabetes.org/DAR
- *African American Program:* diabetes awareness program targeted to the African American community. www.diabetes.org/africanamerican
- *Awakening the Spirit: Pathways to Diabetes Prevention & Control:* diabetes awareness program targeted to the Native American community. www.diabetes.org/awakening

To find out about an important research project regarding type 2 diabetes: www.diabetes.org/ada/research.asp

To obtain information on making a planned gift or charitable bequest: Call 1-888-700-7029. www.diabetes.org/ada/plan.asp

To make a donation or memorial contribution: Call 1-800-342-2383. www.diabetes.org/ada/cont.asp